GLUTEN FREE
SOUL PILOT

Simple and soulful self-care
for the healthy, inspired life you want to live.

Jet Widick *and* Kristen Alden

Gluten Free Soul Pilot

This book presents the research, ideas and experience of its authors and is not intended to be a substitute for consultation with a professional healthcare practitioner. The authors of this book do not dispense medical advice or prescribe the use of any technique as a form of treatment for physical, emotional, or medical issues without the advice of a physician, either directly or indirectly. The intent of the authors is only to offer information of a general nature to help you in your quest for health and well-being. Should you choose to use any of the information in this book for yourself, the publisher and authors assume no responsibility for your actions.

For information about becoming a stockist for Jet Widick's books, please visit the author's website at www.jetwidick.com or email us at wholesale@jetwidick.com.

ISBN 978-0-578-40091-4
First edition, 2018
Printed in the USA

Thank you for your support of independent writers, poets and artists!

calm, not panicked
organized, orderly
beauty, naturally
savory... sweet
that's where the pages meet!

– jet –

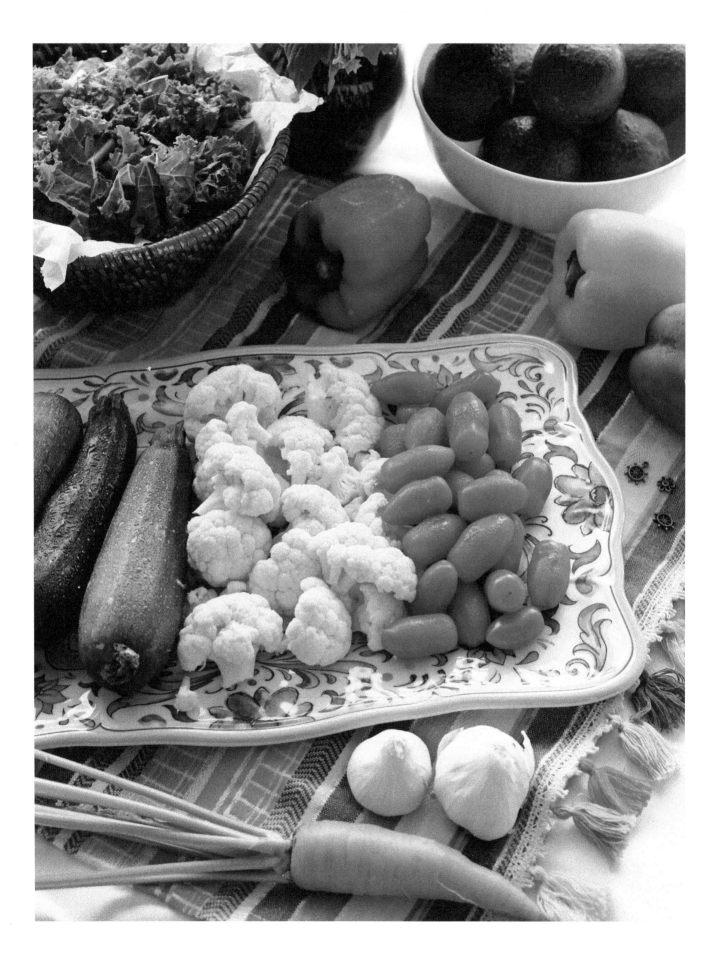

table of contents

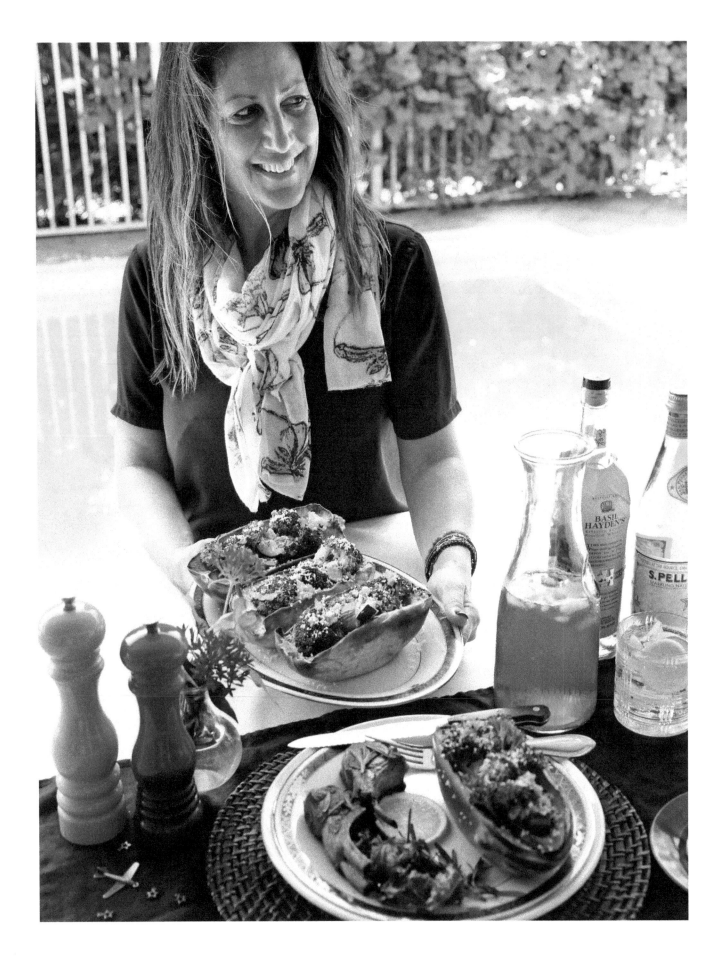

introduction

From Hollywood celebs to Brooklyn bakeries, "gluten-free" may seem like just another buzzword, but—at the beginning of my journey 30 years ago—gluten free hadn't crossed my doctors' minds. I was seriously ill with no diagnoses in sight, and I had no idea that the foods I ate every day were actually killing me.

I was always a skinny kid, so it was hard to know when to worry. I was like any other young gal living off pasta through college and then mac n' cheese once my first son was born. I'm Italian for goodness' sake. Stuffed shells and baked ziti are my specialty! The satisfaction wouldn't last for long, though, and these pasta-filled meals made me feel exhausted. How can a dinner so delicious make a person feel so tired that they can hardly stand?

A year after my first son was born, I realized this was not the food coma fatigue after a big meal. I became severely anemic—and achy. I was dropping weight. My hair was thinning. I was constantly tired and haunted by migraines. I was in bad shape and something needed to change. Turns out, it was my diet.

I'm a nurse and my husband is a doctor, yet it took 15 years of inconclusive tests and feeling unwell to discover that I have celiac disease; an inherited autoimmune disorder that affects the digestive process of the small intestine. In some people with the condition, this results in major gastrointestinal symptoms, including diarrhea, constipation and abdominal pain. But other people with celiac disease don't notice major digestive problems. They may have silent or asymptomatic celiac, characterized by atypical signs and symptoms like fatigue, headaches or joint pain, like myself.

When a person who has celiac disease consumes gluten—a protein found in wheat, rye and barley—their immune system responds by attacking the small intestine and inhibiting the absorption of important nutrients into the body. If undiagnosed and untreated, celiac disease can lead to the development of other autoimmune disorders as well as osteoporosis, infertility, neurological conditions and, in rare cases, cancer.[1]

My story isn't uncommon. And the truth of the matter is that a diagnosis does not equal instant health. The past 15 years living as a diagnosed gluten-intolerant person has had many challenges.

Modern society has made it harder than ever to be healthy. We're confused by all the self-help books, new superfoods, cleanses and eating plans touting that they hold the secret to wellness. We've also become trained to think that health, weight loss and self-care are indulgent, elusive goals that need strict rules and money to be achieved.

The latest trend in health appears to be in elimination diets: watching what you're *not* eating. Based on little or no evidence other than testimonials in the media, people have been switching to gluten-free diets to lose weight, boost energy, treat autism, or generally feel healthier.

In some cases, elimination diets can be very helpful for identifying food intolerances and relieving gastrointestinal upset, irritable bowel syndrome, headaches, and other conditions potentially influenced by diet. For those of us with food allergies and celiac disease, elimination diets are an absolute and life-long requirement. Avoiding certain foods can be a life-or-death matter.

Very often, going gluten-free is mislabeled as a quick-fix, weight-loss diet. Mainstream resources tell us that eating gluten-free is a healthy lifestyle choice. Doctors explain it as the only way to treat newly diagnosed Celiac disease patients—as in my case.

Gluten-free replacement foods are everywhere. They've become synonymous with healthy eating, even for people without celiac disease or gluten intolerance. There may be benefits to a grain-free diet or a low-carb regimen, but the bottom line is that these gluten-free replacements are only substitutions for food that isn't healthy to begin with.

If you're determined to go gluten-free, it's important to know that it can set you up for some nutritional deficiencies. The truth about the "gluten-free diet" is that it's built on the same foundation as the Standard American Diet (SAD). Both are low-fat, highly processed diets made up of too much sugar, too much soy, and what Dr. William Davis refers to as high glycemic "junk carbs".[2]

Four common flours used to replace wheat and gluten are:
- Rice flour (and brown rice flour)
- Potato flour
- Cornstarch
- Tapioca starch

A person diagnosed with celiac already has a severely damaged digestive system and is highly susceptible to poor food choices. If you don't remove the other unhealthy foods contributing to the disease, you're STILL going to end up sick... like I did.[3]

These complicated messages have inaccurately shaped our personal relationship with food and our perceptions on wellness. They compete with our instinctive desire to do something so simple and enjoyable; to eat.

That said, being healthy does not have to be difficult.

Forget restrictive diets, counting calories, macros or estimating point values of food. Let's bring ease and happiness back to our wellness with a simple, easy-to-implement message: food should be nourishing and uplifting—not mentally draining and emotionally discouraging.

So, if this book isn't another fad diet, what is it?

It's a guidebook filled with simple strategies for you to be healthy, so you can spend more of your time and energy on enjoying your life.

I believe there are four principles to consider when on the path to health and healing:

- Finally **Knowing** the cause of what's making you feel bad
- The **Strength** to become the master of your thoughts, diet, fitness and well-being
- The **Wisdom** you gain from your life experiences, lessons, and yes... adversity
- The **Inspiration** you get from being healthy, focused and peaceful

It's important to identify and treat the cause, rather than the symptoms. Walking around with celiac disease or gluten intolerance and not knowing you have it is the equivalent to standing on the center of a seesaw and trying to balance it. You're upright but you're not. You never feel right. You have low energy, an inability to focus, and you feel exhausted.

Health and illness are conditions of the whole individual: physical, spiritual, mental, emotional, genetic, environmental, social and other factors. We must treat the cause by taking all of these factors into account—for both healing and prevention of disease.

This means that the practice of self-care is a necessity, not the occasional indulgence of a spa visit or box of luxurious chocolates as it's often portrayed today. When we spend more time talking about the gratification from high thread count sheets than we do about the benefits of getting enough sleep, we've wandered pretty far from what should be considered healthy for either mind or body.

Self-care isn't just something you do every once in a while when you're feeling overwhelmed. It's what you do every dang day. It's taking care of yourself in a way that doesn't require you to treat yourself in order to restore balance. It's making the commitment to stay healthy and feel good as a regular way of life.

Whether you have celiac or not, these four principles—along with consuming a diet of single ingredient, nutrient dense foods such as vegetables, lentils, beans, nuts, seeds, meats, fish, eggs and fruit—will change your life. It's how we're supposed to live and be at our best. It takes mindful practice not to fall into the trap of a quick meal or a sugar fix, but it also becomes so in "grained" in you that you can't imagine living any other way!

I should note here that I'm not a purist. I enjoy the occasional dessert, pizza slice and tortilla chips at my fave Mexican restaurant. But, I now know that so-called "healthy gluten-free food" can still be processed junk food, and that nutrient-rich, whole foods are where it's at and make me feel GREAT.

Being healthy is easier than you think.

In fact, there are many ways that you can get healthy with minimal effort, and this book will give you the guidance you need to develop your own flight plan and navigate toward creating a life of wellness and inspiration.

Make no mistake: It took me a long time to get here. I've worked hard to learn and focus on how to eat around a food-related illness with the ultimate goal of pure wellness. It worked. I feel better now than I ever have. I finally figured out the balance of diet, exercise and mindfulness that works for me and keeps me energized, happy and—thankfully—healthy.

No matter where you are in your journey, nutrition is never a one-size-fits-all science. Remember that what works for you, may not work for someone else. I urge everyone to remain curious and open-minded, and to take time to learn about health, healing and happiness. Empower yourself.

You will thrive beyond your wildest dreams and it will be worth it.

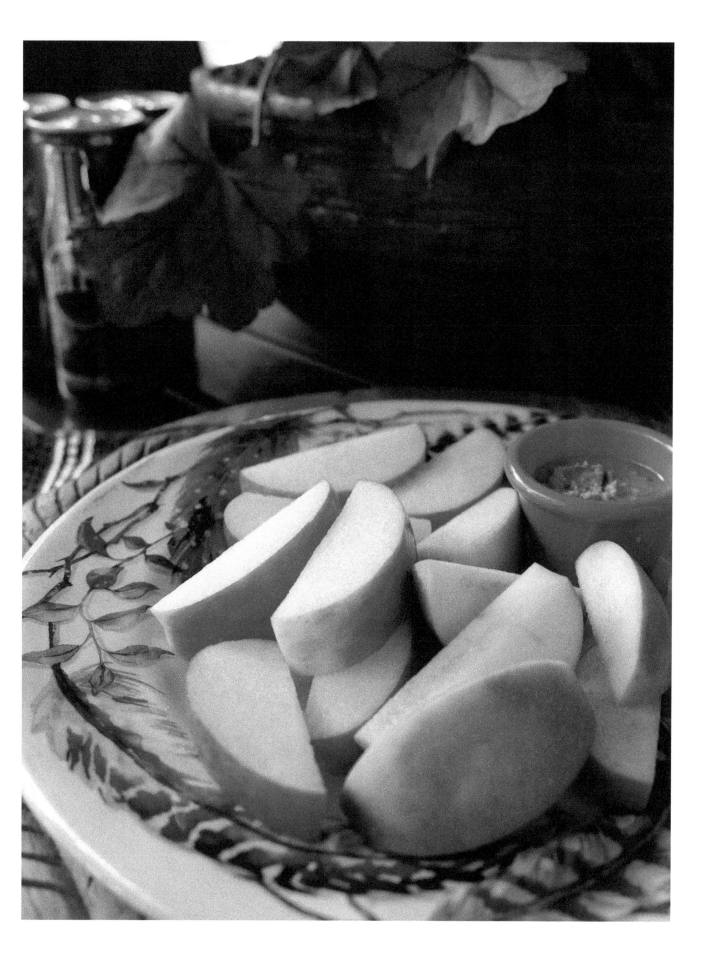

a healthful mission
grounded
no platform needed to stand on
speak it softly, simply
regularly
share it lightly
living brightly
energy from a ray of sunlight
stay steady, a long-lasting program
mind in heart form
wellness
the everlasting aim
everything to gain
daily habits, second nature
keep at it everyday
life changer

– jet –

1

your flight plan

What does it take to take off? To head toward and arrive at pure wellness?

The best way to execute wellness is to design it. Like an architect or a navigator, an explorer or an adventurer, everyone reaching a destination has a plan.

Congratulations on taking the first step on the path to learning to fly! Becoming your own soul pilot will unlock a world of possibilities and give you unparalleled freedom to live in the moment and experience life to the fullest. It is a truly unique experience with wellness as your ultimate adventure. It will be challenging, rewarding and flat out fun!

If you want to create a healthier, simpler and more soulful life, consider building your own personal flight plan. Soul pilot training is a very personal experience, and you'll need to think about how you will learn best and what fits your long-term goals and lifestyle. There is no wrong answer of how to begin. It's important to recognize this as a process; a project that will be adjusted and tweaked along the way, and probably never fully "completed". So, don't overwhelm yourself or put yourself under too much pressure. That will only make you more likely to quit. Focus instead on the long-term benefits of the plan: a better you!

When it comes to success in any type of endeavor, our advice is to take it one step at a time. We are on the move to get better every day, but the truth is we never know exactly where we'll end up. That's why your personal flight plan will focus on the journey, not only the destination.

By focusing on the journey, we don't mean that the destination is not a priority. Having a direction is going to give you a clear goal and clarity of purpose. Why are these important? Because clarity of purpose is the first step to crafting the life you want. Even if you aren't sure yet, you can move into the exploration and experimentation phase of your life and take a self-discovery flight!

"Knowing your why is an important first step in figuring out how to achieve the goals that excite you and create a life you enjoy living (versus merely surviving!). Indeed, only when you know your 'why' will you find the courage to take the risks needed to get ahead, stay motivated when the chips are down, and move your life onto an entirely new, more challenging, and more rewarding trajectory."
-- Margie Warrell, author of *Brave*

We'll reach our destination via Stairsteps—the little increments that help us get to our desired landing place or achieve our goals. And the more we do it, the easier it gets. Self-discovery is a journey. Every new thing we try teaches us a life lesson and gives us yet another experience upon which we rely in order to become ourselves. We carry this learning with us.

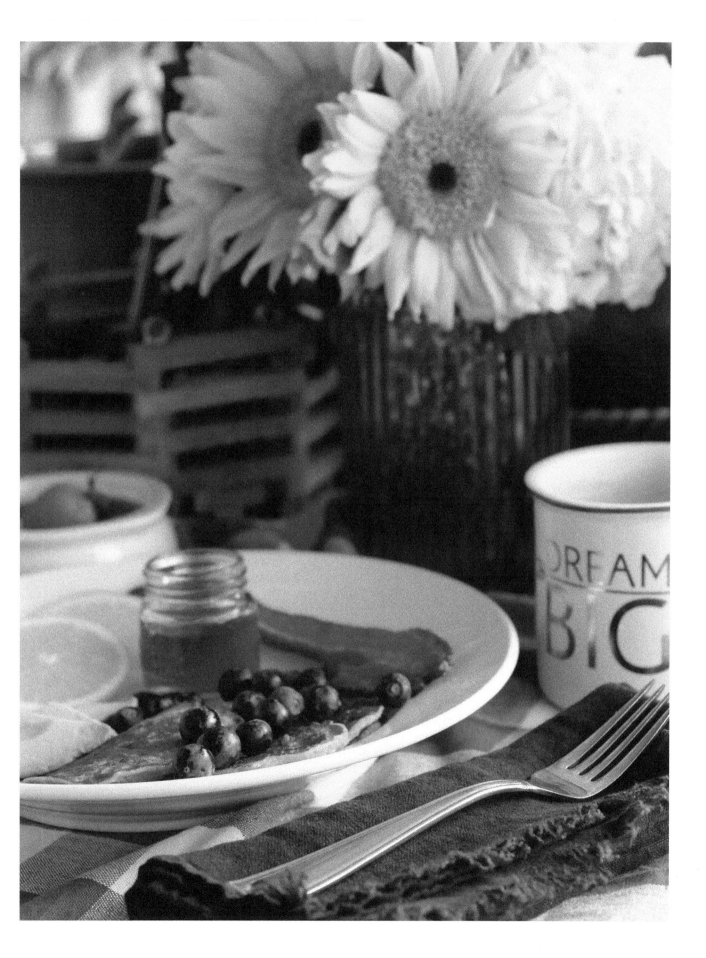

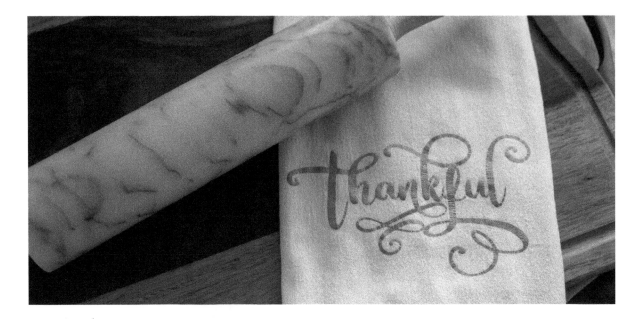

Well-being is everywhere and for everyone. Becoming healthy opened up my world to creativity, and creativity taught me the importance of finding an outlet. Creativity is not exclusive to artistic ability. We're all explorers, students, storytellers, artists, poets and experts in something. And throughout our life, we all become experts in the most important thing of all... our own lives.

Finding that which is best within and sharing it to make the world a more beautiful and joyous place feels alive, expansive and purposeful. Knowing your purpose will unlock your soul gifts, natural talents and creativity to lead you to well-being and living out your highest and most true potential.

You have to rise above your limitations, work to surpass them, and then keep going forward. Don't let yourself be limited by the easy work you've encountered so far. It's tempting to stick with the easy and never try the hard.

A little reminder: **You got this!** Focus on progress, not perfection. Your attitude is a prerequisite for the plan and will point you in the direction of positive growth that is both realistic and achievable. For example, telling yourself *"every moment I'm making an effort to be more mindful about my food choices"* reaffirms that you're closer to the next level up the staircase of your own life and that you have choice in creating a healthier future for yourself.

choose your destination

Remember the *Choose Your Own Adventure* book series from the '80s and '90s where you as the reader assumed the role of the main character and made choices that determined your actions and the plot's outcome? Choosing your destination is fun in a storybook! And yes, you can take part in your own real-life adventure and become the hero of your story.

The rules of the *Choose Your Own Adventure* storybooks are pretty straightforward. You make the choices to guide the plot. Every few pages, you have to make a critical decision on how to proceed. There are many different paths for our stories to take. The beauty is that we get to choose an ending for each path, and making the right choices leads us to the best ending.

Health, healing and happiness don't choose you. These are actual conscious decisions you can make, which can lead you to a storybook life. You decide.

"If you don't know where you are going, you'll end up someplace else."
— Yogi Berra, New York Yankees catcher and manager

As a soul pilot, a flight plan is not optional. It is necessary for having alternate options from takeoff to landing, and for every scenario in between. This will give you an edge and more capacity to deal with the unexpected as the flight unfolds.

To get started, open up a notebook and identify your destination. Be specific. Maybe you want to train 30 minutes a day for your first marathon, or go to bed by 10 p.m. every night so that you can wake up feeling rested and energized. Maybe your goal is to cook three single-ingredient meals at home during the week, or manage your portion sizes by making sure that half of your plate contains vegetables at every meal. Unless you're out for a joyride, you don't just take off and then decide to figure out your destination while en route. Having a definitive wellness vision will guide your expectations and therefore, your results.

Now that you know where you want to go, take a look at what lies between your baseline and the destination. As pilots, we know the simplest and easiest way to travel is in straight lines. Unless terrain, airspace or navigational considerations dictate otherwise, your course should be a straight line from your point of origin to your destination. You'll do this by looking at the big picture of your current health and well-being to establish your wellness baseline, or departure point.

Wellness can be defined as a state of health, yet it extends beyond physical health, nutrition and the number on the scale. Diet, exercise, sleep, self-care, mindfulness, peace and inspiration are all inextricably linked. They cannot be considered separately. Eating healthily, physical activity, a positive outlook, getting rest, and working on inspiring, purposeful projects are all integral to each other for happiness and well-being. It is the balance of an organized whole that is perceived as more than the sum of its parts.

There are two fundamental components to good health:

1. Appropriate treatment for current illness
2. Appropriate preventative care to reduce health decline in the future

While most people actively seek care for current illness, we often forget about the things we can do now for future illness prevention. Your baseline is centered on these two components and has been shaped by your medical, social and family history. It is also constantly being influenced by common factors in your everyday life, such as stress, sleep, exercise and diet.[4]

Our health habits and practices are influenced by many factors, and knowing your personal core values plays a big part in your daily decision making around wellness. It's also a motivator for behavioral change.[5] Do you know your values? Have you ever taken the time to determine what these are? If not, now's the time! Knowing your core values is necessary for the next step: mapping out your preferred flight route between your departure and destination.

Note: Even though you don't have to have perfect health or 20/20 vision to become a soul pilot, it's important to get medical advice before you start. This advice applies to everybody, but in particular to those with pre-existing conditions. For example, celiac disease patients with symptoms of anemia, nutritional deficiencies or weakened bones may require a gentler approach to exercise.

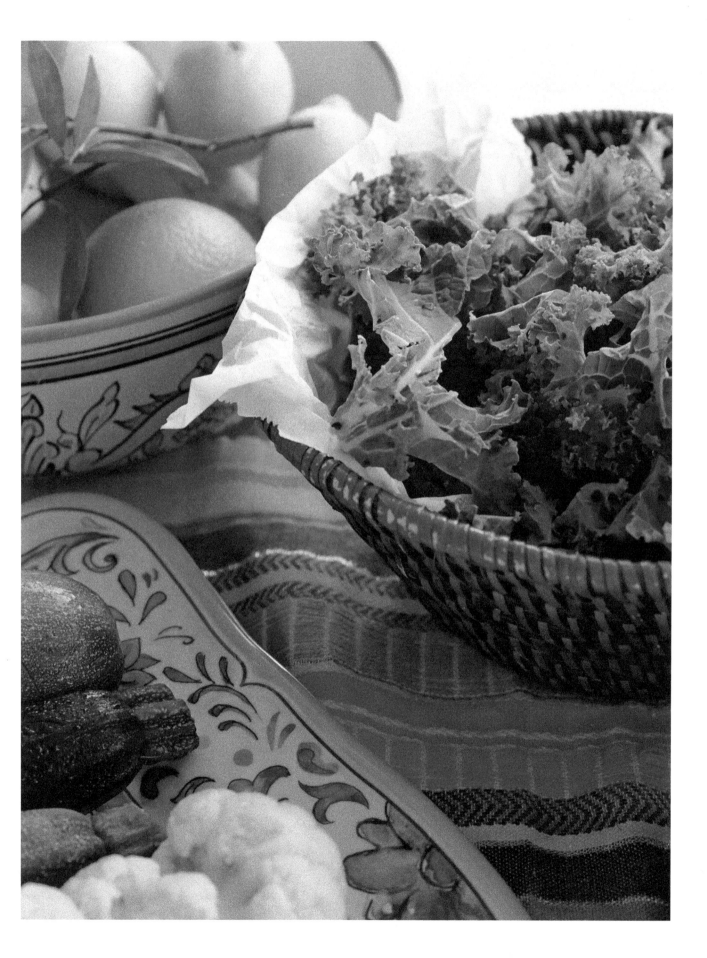

flight route

Choosing your personal values results in clarity and focus, which can greatly streamline your life and your efforts. These priorities will help you determine how to best spend your time and energy. They become your internal reference point for what you believe is good, right and important. Decisions become easier to make.

Whether you are aware of them or not, you have values for every part of your life: parenting values, work values, your values around money, and your health values. Like a compass, our core values keep us on course. Get them right and you'll be swift and focused in your decision making, with clear, forward direction. Leave them ambiguous and you'll be on autopilot heading south, wondering how you ended up off track, concerned and confused.

Most of us don't know our personal values. Instead, we rely upon the values from society, culture and the media. For others, it can take years of soul searching, self-reflection and trial and error to find our core values. We're going to take a direct route, however; one with most headwind, spirit, common sense and smarts.

The route is from A to B. Point A is where you are now—your **wellness baseline**. Point B is your destination—your **wellness goal**. What follows is a values exercise adapted from TapRooT® to help you discover your own personal core values, which will help you create health habits in alignment with what's important to you.[6]

Purpose is about *why* we do what we do, values are *how* we achieve purpose, and habits are *what* we do every day that reflect our purpose and values. Being healthy takes effort and courage. No two people are going to be the same. You might find someone who shares similar desires, interests, and life goals, but ultimately, this is about YOU. Nobody is going to have the exact same values as you. It's not selfish. It's how you achieve a high level of functioning to live your best life.

One of the personal core values at the top of our list, is health. If you have a serious health issue or if your physical health is ever in jeopardy, there are no words to explain how much you care about and respect your well-being, peace, and the ability to feel good every day. I have a great appreciation for waking up with renewed energy and vitality now that I'm well.

1. Determine your personal core values. *From the list below, choose and write down up to 30 core values that resonate with you. Do not overthink your selections. As you read through the list, simply write down the qualities you believe are important. If you think of a value that is personally meaningful and isn't on the list, be sure to write it down as well.*

Abundance	Cooperation	Generosity	Open-minded	Security
Acceptance	Collaboration	Grace	Originality	Self-control
Accountability	Consistency	Happiness	Passion	Selflessness
Achievement	Contribution	Health	Peace	Service
Advancement	Creativity	Honesty	Perfection	Simplicity
Adventure	Credibility	Humility	Performance	Spirituality
Advocacy	Curiosity	Humor	Personal growth	Stability
Ambition	Daring	Inclusiveness	Playfulness	Status
Appreciation	Decisiveness	Independence	Pleasure	Success
Authenticity	Dedication	Individuality	Popularity	Teamwork
Autonomy	Dependability	Influential	Power	Thankfulness
Balance	Diversity	Innovation	Preparedness	Thoughtfulness
Being the best	Empathy	Inspiration	Proactivity	Traditionalism
Benevolence	Empowerment	Intelligence	Professionalism	Trustworthy
Beauty	Encouragement	Intuition	Punctuality	Understanding
Boldness	Enthusiasm	Joy	Quality	Uniqueness
Brilliance	Ethics	Kindness	Recognition	Usefulness
Calmness	Excellence	Knowledge	Relationships	Versatility
Caring	Expressiveness	Leadership	Reliability	Vision
Charity	Fairness	Learning	Resilience	Vitality
Cheerfulness	Family	Love	Resourcefulness	Warmth
Cleverness	Friendships	Loyalty	Responsibility	Wealth
Community	Flexibility	Mindfulness	Responsiveness	Well-being
Commitment	Freedom	Motivation	Risk-taking	Wisdom
Compassion	Fun	Optimism	Safety	Wonder

2. Group all similar values together from the list you just created.

Arrange your 30 values by likeness and similarity. Create a maximum of five groupings and place each word with the group where it makes the most sense to you. See the example below.

Abundance	Beauty	Adventure	Family	Health
Freedom	Creativity	Curiosity	Love	Well-being
Independence	Brilliance	Open-minded	Relationships	Vitality
Flexibility	Excellence	Fun	Happiness	Resilience
Simplicity	Quality	Learning	Joy	
	Inspiration	Intelligence	Kindness	
	Achievement	Passion	Mindfulness	

3. Choose one word within each column that represents the essence of each group of values.
Again, do not overthink your labels. There are no right or wrong answers! You are defining the values that are right for YOU. The words chosen for the example groupings are in bold. Remember, your arrangement may look very different from the one below.

Abundance	Beauty	Adventure	Family	**Health**
Freedom	**Creativity**	Curiosity	Love	Well-being
Independence	Brilliance	Open-minded	Relationships	Vitality
Flexibility	Excellence	**Fun**	**Happiness**	Resilience
Simplicity	Quality	Learning	Joy	
	Inspiration	Intelligence	Kindness	
	Achievement	Passion	Mindfulness	

4. Add a verb to each value.
Write each verb and value out as a sentence so that you can see what it looks like as an actionable core value. For example:

1. Live with independence.
2. Seek opportunities for creativity.
3. Embrace fun.
4. Multiply happiness.
5. Promote health.

Sometimes, the highest priority value of each column will be obvious to you. Other times, you'll have it narrowed down to a few choices, but may have difficulty figuring out which one is the most important among them. When this happens, we recommend that you create a possible scenario for each value and compare these hypothetical situations.

When you create scenarios for the values that are hard to prioritize, the best choice for yourself becomes clear. For example, if you're trying to decide whether adventure or fun is more important to you, ask yourself which you would rather do: go rock climbing or take swing dancing lessons? This suggests that rock climbing would satisfy your value of adventure and swing dancing would satisfy your value of fun—each to around the same degree.

The most important thing you can do for your personal success as a soul pilot is to know your core values, and then use them to guide and lead you. When you need to choose or decide something, you can easily do so by determining if the choice lines up with your true values. A life lined-up with personal values is a well-lived, purpose-filled life!

The amount of years I spent with silent celiac disease took its toll on me and affected my everyday life. Once I went "gluten-free", I had to give careful thought to everything I put in my body. It's a habit that's extremely important to me. I'm committed to paying attention to how different foods make me feel after I eat them. I now know which ones keep me energized, focused and at my best—and stay away from the ones that don't.

Experience has taught me that you don't know where you're going unless you know where you've been—and I recognize the ways in which I never want to physically feel again. Our time is precious. I'm a Lucky Ace to have achieved wellness and am sticking with my personal flight plan, values and routine. Every day it gets easier and easier, and now feels like second nature to me.

"Your beliefs become your thoughts.
Your thoughts become your words.
Your words become your actions.
Your actions become your habits.
Your habits become your values.
Your values become your destiny."
— Mahatma Gandhi, lawyer, politician and Indian civil rights activist

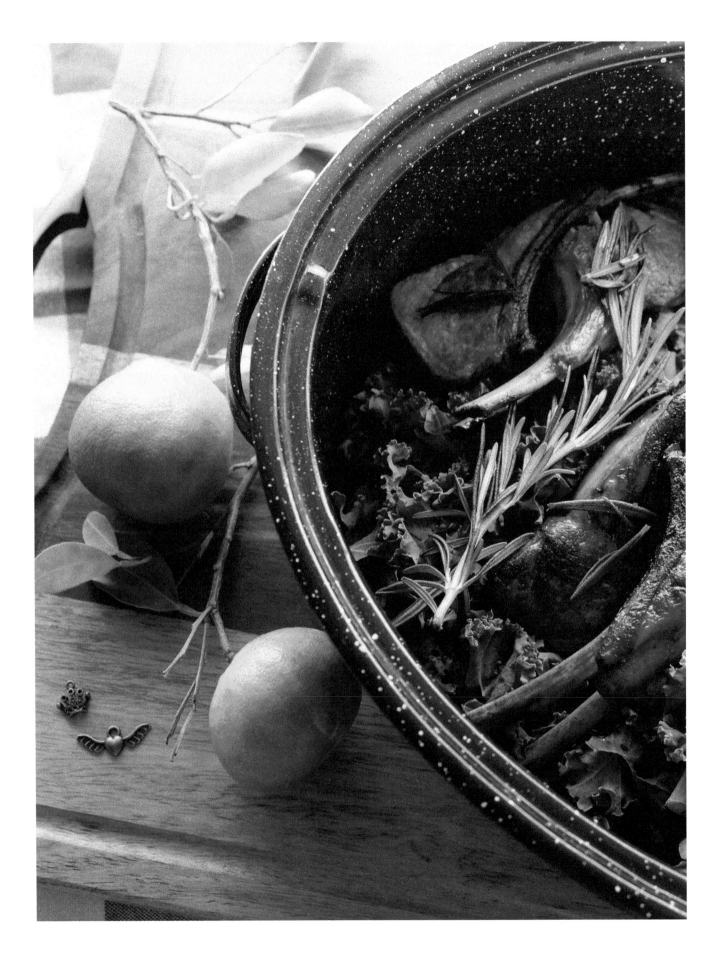

timeline

Now that you've chosen your destination (your specific goal) and determined your flight route (your top five core values), the next step is to come up with a timeline. It's important to remember that it takes time to turn a goal into a habit. How long it takes will depend on a combination of many things, including the behavior itself, your commitment to making the change and your circumstances.

A timeline brings structure and trackability to your goals; keeping you steadily on course so that you'll make it to your destination. Whether it's learning how to cook single-ingredient meals or committing to drinking eight 8-oz. glasses of water every day, any new habit will require a fair amount of energy and time. But if the new behavior doesn't connect with your values, then you'll struggle to create a flight plan that matters to you and becomes a habit.

Healthy habits take smaller, manageable steps to develop. However, if you don't value what you're doing, even the small increments will seem like a pain in the arse. Rather than trying to do something you think you should do, ask yourself, *"What really matters to me?"* Think about how your goal and how you choose to invest your time align with your personal core values.

We suggest a target goal and simple action that YOU choose for yourself. Studies show that progress towards a self-determined behavioral goal supports your feeling of independence and sustains interest, which means that you'll enjoy it more and **keep at it**. There is further evidence that behavior change selected on the basis of personal values, rather than as a way to satisfy external demands (i.e. the need to be skinny), is an easier habit to form.[7]

Habit-formation advice is ultimately simple: Repeat an action consistently in the same context. The purpose here is to select a new action (i.e. eat a piece of fruit in the afternoon) rather than give up an existing behavior (i.e. do not visit the vending machine after lunch) because it's not possible to form a habit for NOT doing something.[8]

"We are what we repeatedly do. Excellence, then, is not an act, but a habit."
— Will Durant, author of *The Story of Philosophy: The Lives and Opinions of the World's Greatest Philosophers*

The popular word on the street is that it takes 21 days to form a new habit, but this turns out to be a myth and isn't backed by any concrete data. Not all habits are created equal and the time it takes for a behavior to become a habit will depend on a variety of different factors, including:

- complexity of the action
- how it fits in your routine
- how often you practice it
- individual differences

Three's a charm is one our favorite things to say, and—according to psychologist and author Jeremy Dean—three months is about how long it will take for a new behavior to become a habit, depending on the above factors. Dean, whose training is in research, explores the science of habits through existing evidence on habit formation.

"The simple answer is that, on average, it took 66 days until a habit was formed. As you might imagine, there was considerable variation in how long habits took to form depending on what people tried to do. People who resolved to drink a glass of water after breakfast were up to maximum automaticity after about 20 days, while those trying to eat a piece of fruit with lunch took at least twice as long to turn it into a habit. The exercise habit proved most tricky with '50 sit-ups after morning coffee,' still not a habit after 84 days for one participant. 'Walking for 10 minutes after breakfast,' though, was turned into a habit after 50 days for another participant."[9]

Everyone is different, so naturally, this will vary based on where you're starting from: your departure point. We all have different wellness ideals. Because of these individual preferences, some of you will travel much farther to your destination than others. Your timeline should reflect what can realistically be accomplished within that time period.

For example, if your goal is to get 12,000 steps in every day and you already walk 10,000 steps a day, this plane is already within sight of its airport and approaching the runway. If your goal is to replace processed foods with fresh, whole foods and you eat frozen, pre-packaged and gluten-free replacement foods at every meal, then your plane is much further away.

It's tempting to pick big, glorious actions when you set out to change a habit, but cool your jets. We're aiming for small, manageable changes until the behavior is in place—then you can scale up. Plus, simpler actions become habitual more quickly and increase self-efficacy. Self-efficacy, or your belief in your own abilities to accomplish a task, plays a major part in how you feel about yourself and whether or not you successfully achieve your goals.[10]

When trying to create new habits, the key is to find or create environmental cues that trigger your new behavior. Psychologist Robert Cialdini offers an easy way of thinking about these triggers by using "if/then" statements.[11] You pick a trigger (if/when) and an action (then). These statements provide a simple formula for taking action that supports your goal.

Value: Happiness
How I want to feel: Energized and joyful
Goal: Exercise for at least 30 minutes most days of the week
When and where: Monday–Thursday mornings at the park
If/then statement(s): When I drop off the kids at school, then I will go for a walk

Value: Achievement
How I want to feel: Focused and productive
Goal: Replace vending machine snacks with fruit
When and where: Weekday afternoons at the office
If/then statement(s): If I get hungry after lunch, then I will eat an apple and drink water

Daily habits are how we live out our purpose and put values into practice. Creating these plans in advance makes it easier to follow through on them. Some people find it helpful to keep a record while they are forming a new habit. The exercise below can be used until your new habit becomes automatic, and the tick sheet on the next page will help you track your progress. Rate how automatic it feels at the end of each week, to see how it gets easier over time.

1. Decide on a goal you would like to achieve for your health and well-being that aligns with your personal core values.

2. Choose a simple action that you can do on a consistent or daily basis to get you toward your goal.

3. Plan when and where you will do your chosen action. Choose a time and place that you encounter regularly throughout the week.

4. Every time you encounter that time and place, do the action.

5. Understand that there will be some resistance during the growth spurt, and it will get easier with time. By 12 weeks you should find that you are doing it automatically without even having to think about it.

6. Congratulations! *If* you made through until the end, *then* you've made a healthy habit!

Keeping track of your progress:

Fill in this tick sheet every day to record how things are going and help you stay focused.

	m	t	w	th	f	s	s	How many days of the week does your action take place?	How automatic does it feel? Rate from 1 (not at all) to 10 (completely).
week 1									
week 2									
week 3									
week 4									
week 5									
week 6									
week 7									
week 8									
week 9									
week 10									
week 11									
week 12									

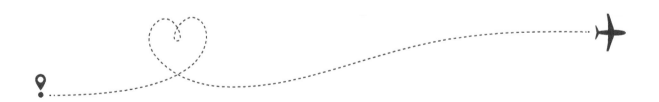

inspiration conversation
without reservation
from someone with an incredible reason
for celebration
healthy route gratification
one day at a time declaration

– jet –

fuel calculation

There are few "diet" books that address eating and feeding your soul as a spiritual practice, but as soul pilots, we're committed to happiness over weight loss metrics or numbers on a scale. The most important thing to us is how we want to feel every day. Behind every goal—every desire—there is a feeling. Your feelings will be the fuel that lead you to your destination.

What gets you up in the morning? What fuels you? For us, it's desire. It's inspiration. Those are the sparks that ignite *everything*.

An often overlooked and incredibly important aspect of finding what pushes our buttons is the need to be well. We can't schedule inspiration or force it into existence, so we have to create a favorable environment to receive it. When you nourish your body, you feed your soul. And, being strong and healthy will open your world up to desire and inspiration—both which transform the way we perceive our own capabilities.

How do you want to feel in your body? Do you want to feel strong? Beautiful? Loved? Energized? Confident? Balanced?

To experience the way you want to feel, you'll need to do simple and practical things on a daily basis that will help you feel that way. The purpose here is to seek out the environments and activities that overlap your personal core values and make decisions that align with your desired feelings.

Once you get clear on how you want to feel, it's time to pay attention and listen to what your body is telling you. Our emotions are valuable sources of information. They give us direction and help us understand what we need.

Listening to your feelings doesn't mean following them impulsively or blindly. Part of the essence of being a soul pilot in command of your aircraft *(your being)* means realizing the fact that: 1) you're on your own in your decision making, and 2) others aboard are depending on you. Of course, you aren't completely on your own—as you'll have resources like air traffic control *(your tribe)*, and perhaps a co-pilot *(your partner)*—but ultimately, you're the one in control and navigating your options. You get to choose.

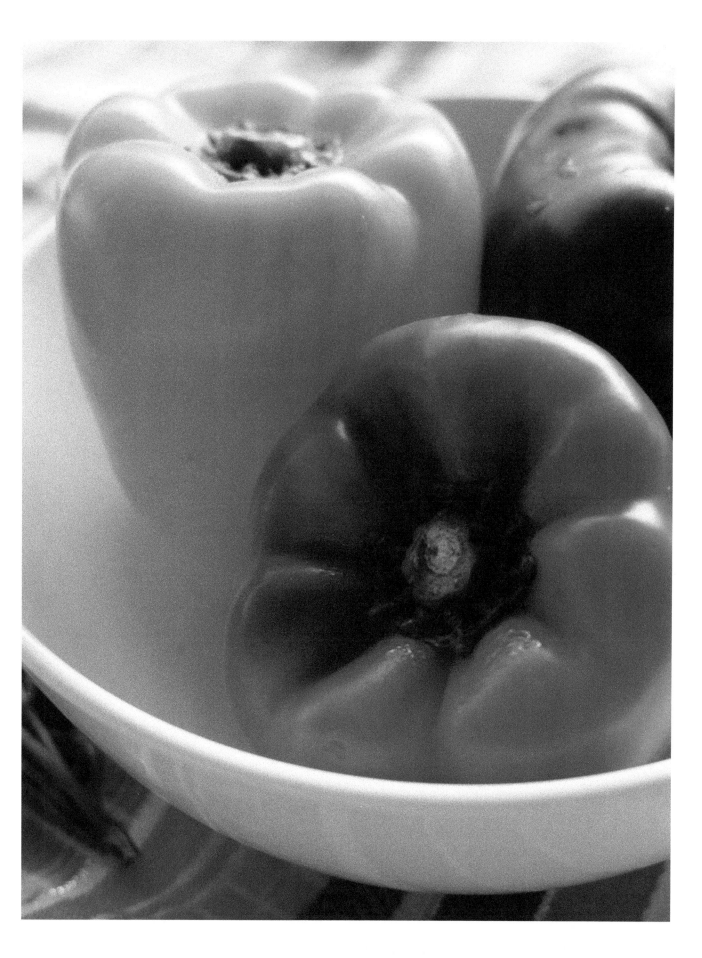

On every journey there comes a moment when we wish we had a little more fuel. Perhaps the headwind was stronger than forecast. Maybe you took a detour around some bad weather. It could be that the gauges dropped sooner than you hoped they would, or your planning could've been better. Whatever the reason, you find yourself in that discouraging spot: a certain distance from your destination—unsure if you'll crash short of the runway.

Fuel management is part of Aviation 101, which every soul pilot needs to know from the beginning. We pay particular attention to our energy reserves and stress that running out of fuel happens way too often for any of us to get comfortable with the idea that it'll never happen. Running out of gas is something you can avoid with proper planning and mindful decision making.

Your fuel calculations will be based on:

1. **Premium fuel**
2. **Straight route**
3. **Steady speed**
4. **Properly tuned engine**

There is no more obvious way to save fuel than to travel a shorter distance, which is why you'll plan your route accordingly. Our emotions are our personal GPS route planner. Call it intuition, your gut feeling, a sixth sense... your internal compass exists to help guide you. If we program a destination into it, its job is to instruct us step by step on how to get there and to let us know if we're staying on- or getting off-course.

There are so many people who don't know what they're eating. They're not aware of the inferior quality of much of the food in the United States, and—even when informed—resist changing their eating habits. One of the most important aspects of owning your sacred aircraft is properly taking care of it. While regular maintenance is certainly important, do you put much thought into the fuel you use to keep moving forward?

Emotions are the raw material of our desires, needs and hopes. In order to gauge your route from your emotions, you must first understand why you eat certain things and how the food you eat matters to your well-being. Premium fuel is the best choice when it comes to our bodies.

Stocking up on inferior products and then eating these processed foods when you come home drained from an exhausting day at work is problematic. When we regularly miss out on sleep to pack as much as we can into our lives, it leaves us feeling stressed and tired—which also makes it harder to resist high-calorie, nutrient-empty foods throughout the day.[12]

Processed foods have become a well-established part of our diets, but much of the packaged foods you'll find at the grocery store contain empty calories. This means they contain little or no essential vitamins or minerals. In other words, these foods provide nothing of value to your body.[13]

When someone is in a bad mood, why will they choose to eat junk food? And when someone is in a good mood, why will they make healthier food choices? To get at the why, Cornell University did a study on how people react to their moods and emotions and the perspective of time to explain food choice. Basically, when we feel uncomfortable or are in a bad mood, we focus on what is close and convenient, which gets us to focus more on the immediate sensory qualities of our foods—like how it tastes and smells, as well as its mouthfeel and texture. When we're in a good mood and things seem okay, then we're able to take a big picture perspective. This kind of thinking allows us to focus on the more abstract aspects of food, including how healthy it is.[14]

Evoking a multi-sensory experience through food creates a pleasurable experience, and food scientists within the processed food industry know this. For example, at Tasty Bite, a maker of Indian and Asian microwavable entrees, a trained, discriminating sensory panel considers five food attributes when developing something new: color/appearance, texture, taste, aroma and flavor. Products must register high on the panel's "wow meter" in order to pass the test.[15]

So many of us feed our feelings, which can put us into a tailspin.

When you are able to pinpoint the emotions behind your food choices and the trigger foods that fuel your unhealthy cravings, then you get straight to the heart of the matter. You streamline your thinking down to the essence and can make decisions around your needs. You stay focused and strong in moments of challenge.

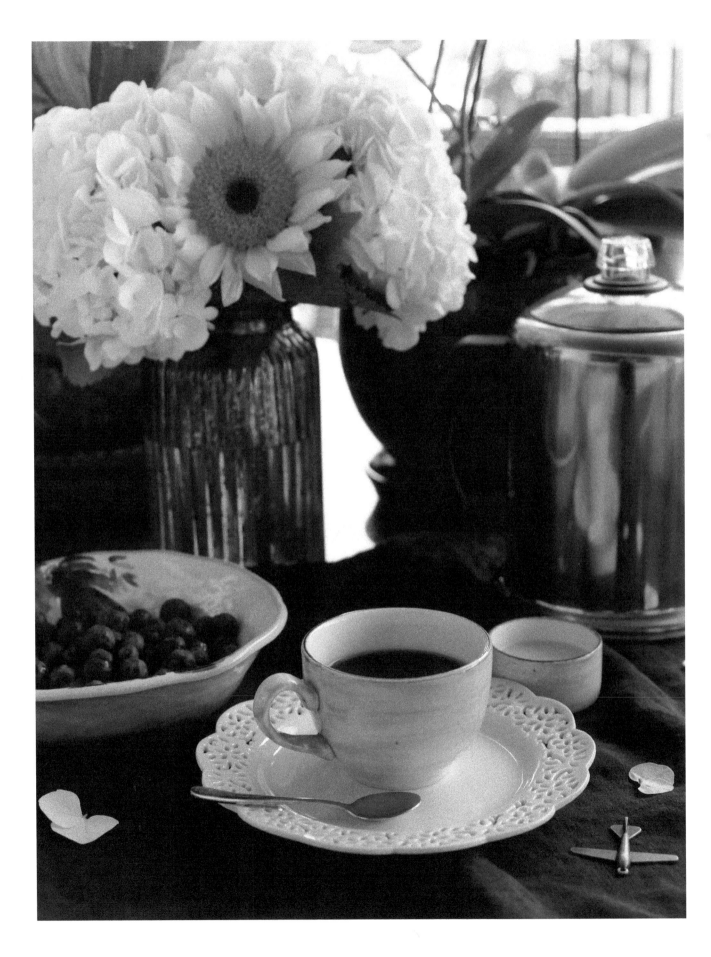

Inspiration and desire come from the heart. When working toward a meaningful goal that aligns with your values, temptations and discouragements may hit you, but they won't stop you. Your emotional GPS will recalibrate and direct you back on track.

"From time to time, you may stumble, fall. You will for sure—count on this, no doubt—you will have questions and you will have doubts about your path. But I know this: If you're willing to listen to and be guided by that still small voice that is the GPS within yourself, to find out what makes you come alive, you will be more than okay. You will be happy, you will be successful, and you will make a difference in the world."
— Oprah Winfrey, media executive, talk show host, actress, producer and philanthropist

Once you've course corrected, you can begin to build a steady momentum. A steady flight is best to maximize your fuel efficiency, and soul pilots know the fastest way to move forward in life is to go slow. There's a reason supersonic planes didn't become an everyday vehicle. If you slow down your speed, your resistance decreases, which means more comfort for you and your passengers. Takeoffs and landings are much simpler and softer. Your aircraft also won't wear-out as quickly.

Slowing down to go fast may sound counterintuitive, but greatness takes time. Building an exceptional life takes time. Developing excellent habits that make you an amazing human being take *time*. When you slow down, you create the space for grace—the place where your full attention intersects with the present moment. And when you create the space for grace, you tap into your intuition, inspiration and intention.

Play the long game, be patient and go at a sustainable pace. Do less. Disconnect from technology. Focus on people. Go for a walk. Breathe deeply. Eat slowly. Learning to be fully present connects you to your body so you can nourish it with exactly what it needs.

Distractions are everywhere, waiting to lead us down the wrong path. Deciding what to subtract from your life is one of the key components to steadiness. Slowing down allows you to focus your attention on the main markers of your behaviors throughout the day, such as an unhealthy breakfast on your way to work, taking the elevator instead of the stairs or having a drink in front of the TV when you get home. These habits structure your day and set the tone for your general decision-making preferences, whether they serve your highest potential or not.

Changing a habit isn't easy. It's likely to involve a fair amount of discomfort in the beginning. But, the best part of disrupting an ingrained habit is that it makes new room for a good habit to go in its place.

"Perfection is achieved, not when there is nothing more to add, but when there is nothing left to take away."
— Antoine de Saint-Exupéry, poet, pilot and author of *The Little Prince*

Maintaining a steady flight requires a balance, described as the equilibrium of all the forces acting upon the aircraft. We often find that balance requires us to move toward the opposite of our usual habits and comfort zones. For many of us, this means learning how to *yield*. When applying this to practice, we try to strike that balance between **effort** and **ease**. This is when we exert enough effort to be steady and strong, but with enough ease to remain comfortable.

Effort: We find a way to show up every day in light of any limitations or obligations we may have. We don't say one thing and do another. Instead, we show up for the people in our lives and for ourselves. We stand strong for what we believe in and what's important to us.

Ease: We first make time to create a space of ease through preparation and planning. We create a place that is soft and feels good. Ease dissuades us from pushing too hard, while at the same time, encourages us not to run away.

True wellness is not waiting to get healthy. It's creating the environment where health and wellness take place. Your motivation is sparked by a deep desire within you that sets things in motion. How you fuel your motivation will determine if you reach your destination. Whatever your goals may be, they need to be nurtured to their fullest potential through the engine of inspired action.

The difference between inspired action and forced action is critical to keeping a finely tuned engine. Forced action is action taken for the sole purpose of trying to make something happen. It's action you take because you think you "should" be doing something. You can tell when you're doing this type of action because there is little to no excitement and motivation. Your engine is moving and acting and doing and working, but not much seems to be happening. You're spinning your engine and getting nowhere.

In contrast, inspired action comes from an internal desire to do something. It's the action you take when your soul says, "YES!" This type of action is almost always accompanied by a rush of excitement, enthusiasm and joy. When your engine of inspiration is running, you are in the zone and flying along at a cruising altitude. Everything flows. You may work harder, but it doesn't always feel like work.

We know we need motivation to keep us moving forward, but pay particular attention to the reasons and incentives behind it. What is pushing you? What is pulling you?

Forced action is your push. Push motivation comes from a desire to make a change away from an undesired state. It's the type of motivation required from you to complete a task where the end goal is the most important thing, and the means to reach it don't matter so much. This type of action will initially get you off the ground. However, thoughts and feelings directed toward pushing away from things you *don't* like won't keep you airborne for long. The extra baggage puts too much wear and tear on your engine.

Inspired action is your pull, and a quieter, more fuel-efficient mode of propulsion. Pull motivation is not generated by external forces such as guilt or fear, but comes from within yourself and is built on a desire to better your life. This type of action is a renewable source of energy and can be used to achieve additional range. You'll also enjoy the journey so much that—not only will you reach your end goal—you'll want to keep going above and beyond your original destination.

The main difference between the two is that push motivation is typically linked to negative emotions (working toward not feeling bad about yourself), and pull motivation is coupled with the positive ones (envisioning a happier, thriving version of yourself). While both have their place along your path, pull motivation is best for establishing long-term change.[16]

"Follow the pull. It's the first step toward flying."
— Danielle LaPorte, entrepreneur, poet and author of *The Firestarter Sessions*

Whenever you're feeling the push, it may be time to check-in for fine-tuning and preventative maintenance. Similar to Momma Annabelle's special recipe variation of chicken parmesan, this engine tuning requires personalized tweaking to take it from a basic, out-of-the-box "heat-and-serve" adjustment to something unique and optimized for your personal aircraft. This process requires love, patience, attention to detail, and a dash of creative flare. The good news is that there are many tools easily accessible to you to help with this task—and most of them are already installed from the factory.

core values
as your takeoff place
pure wellness
at your own pace
slow and steady
it's not a race
love you as you
and that pretty face
keep the smile
walk the mile
don't stop
it's worth the while

– jet –

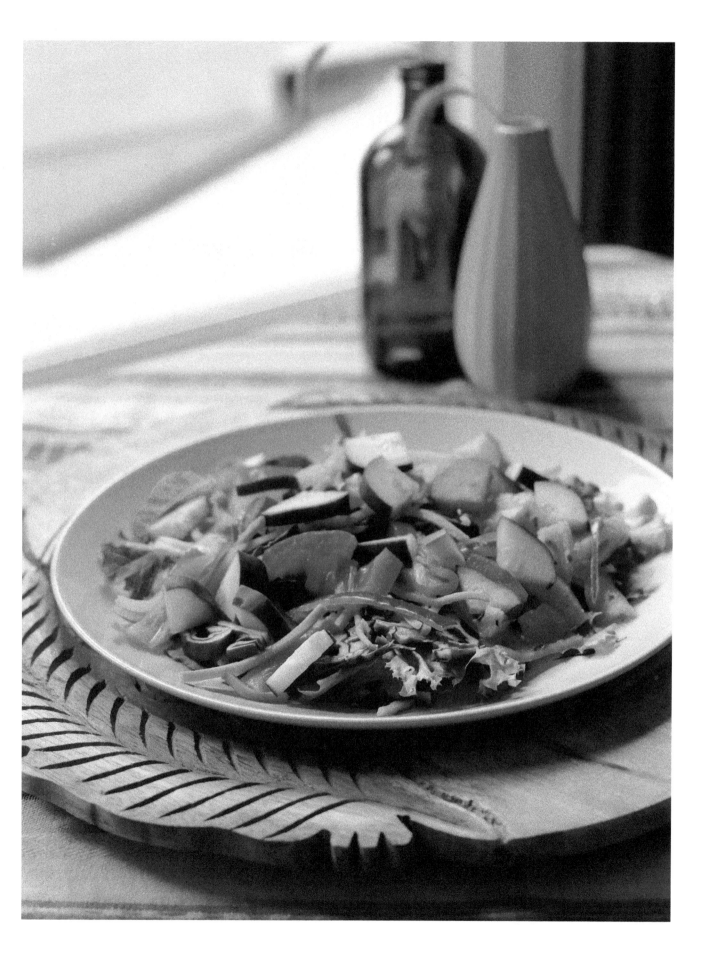

air traffic compliance

When it comes to health and wellness, there is no cookie-cutter plan that will work for everyone. The key is to find out what works for YOU and then stay out of your own way once you set out to achieve your goal. For many of us, the mental aspect is much more challenging than the actual physical work required to reach our destination.

The success of your flight relies on a calm, controlled flight deck. When you show up to work, you have to have a set of rules and standards in place for all phases of the journey.

The main objective of Air Traffic Compliance in particular is to enhance your pull motivation and therefore, your ability to meet your goals. This is achieved by establishing and monitoring three things to provide a fulfilling experience to satisfy both your needs and expectations:

1. **Standards** (Quality Control)
2. **Mindset** (Quality Assurance)
3. **Integrity** (Standard Operating Procedures)

Compliance gets a bad rap because it's immediately associated with constraints or punishment for not following the rules. Soul pilot compliance, however, has nothing to do with either. Ours is a self-compliance to our personal values and a life-affirming platform for being. It's a supervitamin for the spirit and a structure that can set you free.

High standards are a source of your competitive advantage with respect to yourself, and are essential to achieving your goals. High levels of quality are therefore not an added value, but a basic requirement. The quality doesn't relate solely to your end goal either, but also to the way you do your work and show up every day.

Your current standards originate from your environment, what people teach you and your personal beliefs. These standards are the reference points you use to determine whether an action is appropriate or desirable, meaning, whether you should do it or not.

"Work is love made visible."
— Kahlil Gibran, poet, artist and author of *The Prophet*

It's easy to get caught-up in the idea that hard work and labor are a burden, rather than viewing both as a playing field for us to develop our highest potentials and experience new perspectives. But, it's what our work represents and ultimately allows us to do and be—which is to make visible to those in our lives how much we love, care, and support them, as well as ourselves.

Our actions and efforts—with no guarantee of reward—can feel risky; like a futile quest through the clouds. But when you think about it, all that we do in our lives is work. Some may call it play, but that's just a different kind of work (working on oneself to be healthy, feel well, be happy, be a better musician, write poetry, etc.).

Work gets us in touch with our personal core values. It connects us with others in meaningful ways. It provides us with a platform to contribute our unique gifts and recognize our own strengths. Through our work we get to know ourselves better, while experiencing the benefits of tangible results. And, our purpose is matched by the effort we're willing to put forth on its behalf.

It's important to go after the things you care about and value. When you do, it'll bring you closer to your truth. Soul piloting is a labor of love. We know the process affects the outcome and that there's more fulfillment at the next level up our life's elevation. When we take on our dreams and desires with our whole heart, this whole-heartedness leads to a result we can love and appreciate.

When we love, we strive to become better than we are. I find encouragement in these words whenever trying something new.

"It is we who nourish the Soul of the World, and the world we live in will be either better or worse, depending on whether we become better or worse."
– Paulo Coelho, author of *The Alchemist*

If standards focus on fulfilling quality requirements, then mindset provides confidence that those requirements are met. This mentality must align with your values and purpose, as your commitment and active involvement are essential for ensuring how appropriate and effective your beliefs are to your desired outcome.

Your mindset serves as a passport to your success by giving you greater control, which allows you to more easily plan and predict. Remember atmospheric conditions can change and the weather on which you base your flight plan is only forecasted and not exact. You must be prepared to make continual course corrections. Just as an aircraft faces headwinds, downdrafts, storm fronts, wind shear and unexpected turbulence, you will experience the same in the pursuit of any worthwhile goal.

However, when things get bumpy—like navigating through a thunderstorm—you divert your focus to stay in control. This is done through understanding how you react to stress and deciding what you want from the situation. Be aware of how you're feeling and commit to keeping cool under pressure. Determine to get to the root cause of the situation before allowing yourself to make conclusions or pass judgment. A walk outside, some fresh air, listening to music, deep breaths, meditation and mindfulness are all easy, doable solutions to keep calm. Remember that life is happening *for* you, not *to* you.

Unfortunately, once we take a quick break, reality is right in front of us again. So, what do you do to stay on your flight plan? Show yourself some appreciation and compassion. We mistakenly believe that being hard on ourselves is the only way to stay on course, but science shows that being kinder is actually the secret to greater motivation; that it won't just help you feel better, it will also help you perform better.[17]

The number one reason people give for not being self-compassionate is that they're afraid they will let themselves get away with anything if they're too soft on themselves. They believe their internal judge plays a crucial role in keeping them in line and on track. In other words, they confuse self-compassion with self-indulgence.[18]

According to self-compassion researcher and author Dr. Kristin Neff, self-compassion has been shown to increase people's motivation to learn, to change for the better and to avoid repeating past mistakes. Self-compassion increases people's capacity for creativity and curiosity. In addition, self-compassionate people tend to have high personal standards and are more likely to take risks. They have less fear of failure and show greater confidence in their abilities to reach their goals. And if they don't meet those goals, they're not as upset about inevitable aspects of work and life. People who practice self-compassion also tend to have more intrinsic motivation and don't need as many external rewards in order to move toward their goals.[19]

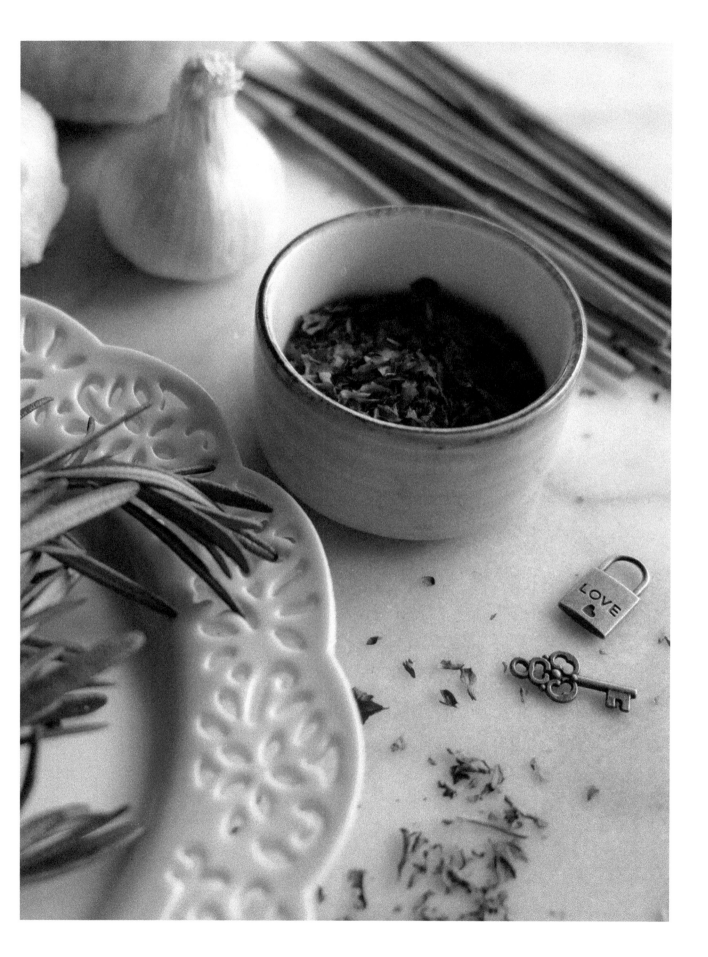

"Whether you think you can or think you can't—you're right."
– Henry Ford, founder of the Ford Motor Company

Mindset is the single most important factor in stabilizing our challenges. Mental training can help you learn how to control your thoughts so that they no longer consume you and hold you back from reaching your goals, but instead fuel positive action and nurture a most confident, focused, and enhanced version of YOU.

From the earliest days of flight training, pilots are taught an important set of priorities that should follow them through their entire flying career: aviate, navigate and communicate. The top priority—always—is to fly the aircraft first. To a Soul Pilot, following this simple phrase can mean the difference between victor or victim.

It's a very simple principle and means you only need to focus on the single, closest and most critical issue. Once that's solved, you can move on to the next. If you think about all the factors that influence your life on a daily basis, which is the most pressing and immediate in terms of your health and wellness? By addressing the most immediate need or concern, you're able to diffuse the situation enough to find the space and time to assess the next priority. Some turbulence may not even exist at all—other than in your mind—but the tangible thing that threatens your well-being the most is the one you address on the first step towards your destination.

For example, the foremost issue could be a matter of making yourself a priority and carving out time in your week to go to yoga or get outside for a brisk walk. Once you make the commitment to yourself in this way, the follow-up becomes the next obstacle. That is to say, how you perceive your fulfillment of this commitment can either be reinforcing or discouraging. If you're only able to go to yoga or walk twice a week, but promised yourself three, then you have a choice: 1) Give yourself props for going twice (which is more than you were doing), or 2) Criticize yourself for not fulfilling your promise.

If we divert our attention to the one circumstance that negatively triggers us, the positive areas in our life will suffer.[20] You can choose to not believe in thoughts that don't serve your well-being or that influence your life in a negative way. These are styles of thinking like catastrophizing, over-generalizing, blaming and discounting the positive.[21] Let the trigger for this mindset be the identification of the thought, and therefore, false. When a non-serving thought manifests, notice it and say to yourself, "I don't believe it."

How you choose to feel about your results will either propel you forward into greater balance and wellness or send you into a nosedive. It's your choice. Once you become aware of how your beliefs affect your behavior, your behavior and habits will follow. When you let go of the false belief that you are lacking or inadequate, in that moment, you arouse your potential. You empower yourself to make the next critical decision for greater health and happiness with clarity and perspective.

"The irony is that we attempt to disown our difficult stories to appear more whole or more acceptable, but our wholeness—even our wholeheartedness—actually depends on the integration of all our experiences, including the falls."
– Brené Brown, research professor and author of *Rising Strong*

Thinking positively has its benefits, no doubt, but thinking *authentically* has even more to commend. To be authentic is to be whole; to acknowledge that the richness of life lies in its contrasts—its light and shade—and in our capacity to feel and acknowledge the full spectrum of our experience.

If you flew the airplane perfectly all the time, none of this would be of any concern to you. But, the system includes more than just you. You have to fly in an unpredictable environment, with other less-than-perfect airplanes sharing your airspace, and in a system with rules that can vary from place to place and change from day to day. Perfection is impossible.

Your integrity is your standard operating procedures and the cornerstone of smooth operations in an ever-changing landscape. Integrity is defined as consistency of actions, values, methods, measures, principles, expectations, and therefore, outcomes. Integrity helps us stay on course without colliding with our personal core values, while also regulating and guiding us to our arrival point. Putting a set of procedures in place is thus something that is very expansive and covers all areas into which aircraft venture.

To have integrity is to be authentic—whole and undivided—and is a practice we commit to every day. If we say we believe something but actually believe something different, or if we say we're going to do something but actually do something else, then we create conflict within ourselves. Our commitment—our word—begins to lose value and affect our quality of life. We become divided, and small cracks in our integrity over time will eventually weaken our aircraft.

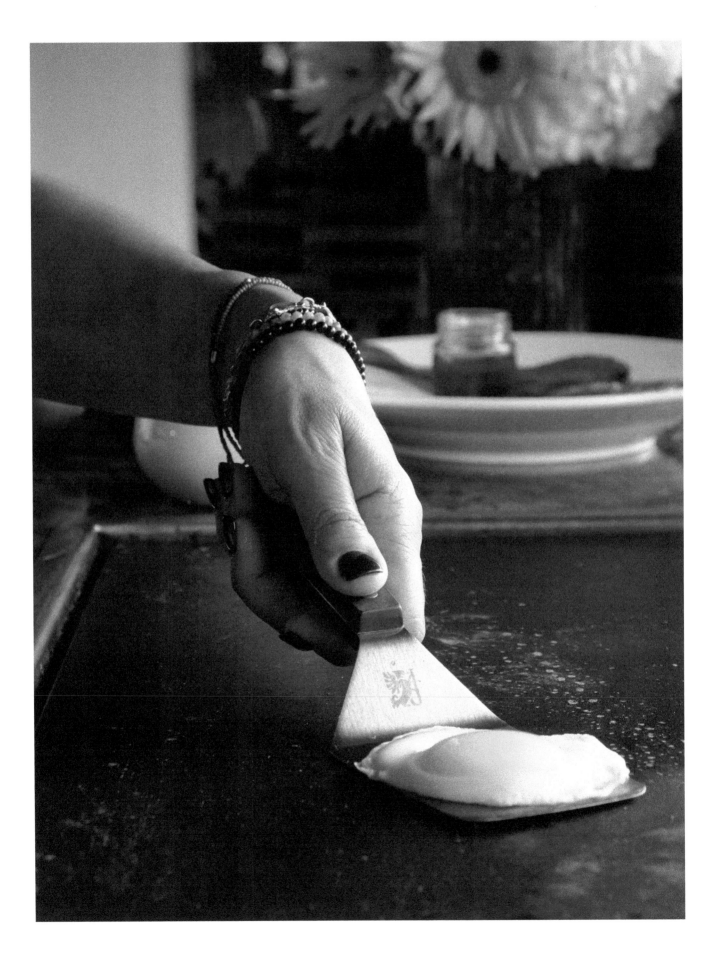

One reason for our lack of commitment could be that there are no established standards to follow. When there are no standards, our actions are based on personal judgment and a lot of guesswork. The inevitable consequence of this is confusion, stress and dissatisfaction. However, the solution is never to work harder at covering mistakes. The key is to work smarter. Integrity makes this happen.

"Trust yourself. Create the kind of self that you will be happy to live with all your life."
– Golda Meir, labor Zionist leader, diplomat and Israel's fourth Prime Minister

Like the processes and standards the business world must follow, your unique set of principles provide focus and direction for soul piloting this eternally great, unfathomable and infinite life around you. With standards, you can create the sacred space you need to look out for yourself and adjust when needed. Adherence to standards and processes can actually provide a level of freedom and flexibility because your mental and physical well-being will eventually become more predictable.[22]

Meals adhere to balanced compliance. You show up at the gym because you have a schedule. Health is maintained because you stick to a routine. Goals are hit because you turn the pages over in your planner and draw a butterfly as each day is completed. We create high standards because it gives us a sense of pride and accomplishment. And once you have pride and accomplishment that comes from a place of love—the most important ingredient in life next to air—you'll have the desire and discipline to go the distance.

Every action begins with a decision. Before you get started on creating standards on which to base your journey, you'll need to identify the mindset in which you perform your best and the routes that encourage you to create that ideal environment. Write it down. Come up with your own personal mission statement. How will you practically and authentically apply this to your daily life?

It's easy to get caught up in the moment and forget why you have these processes in place. Bottom line, we have them because they maximize our investment in the short time we have on this planet. By upholding your standards and following your guidelines, you can create the healthy, inspired life you want to live. Choice by choice. Day by day. It may take longer than you'd like, but this is the making of a good life. **And if it's worth having, then it's definitely worth working toward.**

pay attention to your flight path
follow your call to adventure—do the math
how does it add up?
your True North
plus this moment together
a goal to keep at it
making life better
stay on track to your destination
with courage, no hesitation
it's simple
make it your very own
you'll reach arrival
flying straight to your heart's home
celebrating the beautiful victories
no stopping
the rest is history

— jet —

arrival

To successfully navigate your aircraft to arrival, it's important to understand which way is north. There are two norths you'll need to consider, and which one you choose has critical implications upon where you'll end up.

So, just what are these two norths? First, there's True North, which is your internal compass in relation to where you are now. This north represents who you are at your essence and how you live and love from your personal core values. The second north—magnetic north—is the external world, which is constantly (and quite rapidly) moving. Soul pilots use True North for their orientation. It keeps us grounded even though we are flying high.

When our compass is pointed toward True North, we are mindful and our souls are calm and peaceful. On this path, we have the capacity to listen to our hearts and stay in touch with what's meaningful to us. Our True North gives us the ability to *respond* from our conscious values and not *react* from our subconscious autopilot. Our core values determine the beliefs we hold about ourselves and the direction our lives will take. When they aren't carefully vetted, we end up at the whims of our environment from an amalgamation of subconscious thoughts and habits.

When we're flying on autopilot, we risk falling into conditioned patterns of thought and behavior, most of which we did not consciously choose and was handed down to us from our culture and upbringing. Living in unawareness like this can lead to a sense of discontent and disconnection from ourselves when not aligned with our personal core values.

Magnetic north is a life created by default, whereas True North is a life created by design. A life created by design is a journey toward higher expression of yourself, toward the kind of person you know in your heart you came here to be. And as all journeys, it begins when you make the conscious choice or commitment to follow the call to adventure from within your soul.

"I have learned that as long as I hold fast to my beliefs and values—and follow my own moral compass—then the only expectations I need to live up to are my own."
– Michelle Obama, lawyer, writer and former First Lady of the United States of America

Two norths would be more of an interesting bit of trivia than an essential navigation factor if the two poles resided in the same location, however they do not align. And if the two norths weren't enough of a nuisance for a soul pilot in training, there's another issue: the magnetic field drifts, which causes the location of magnetic north to change over time. This in turn means the angle of variation between magnetic north and your True North varies from place to place and shifts over time, too.

So, what does all this mean to you?

Do not be discouraged by what you cannot see. Your journey is not a linear process. It may seem as if nothing is happening on the surface, or that your goals are progressing slowly, but that does not equal defeat. It is progress, however slow it may be, because you are moving forward toward your goals and desires. Your journey is about the transformation that takes place within and over a series of adaptations—with your intention to improve the quality of your life.

When you are acting in alignment with your True North, there may be an initial period of awkwardness, as there is with anything new. Your authentic self is a sum of many parts that will come to you bit by bit until you've found enough to feel whole. Enough to know what makes you feel good. Enough to know where moments of hope and happiness can be found. Enough to know that you are on the authentic path for YOU.

Let your imagination soar and hold nothing back. Remember that your compass is there to help guide you to arrival—but is not the territory. Progress is impossible without change.

Throughout our lives we will come across moments disguised as challenges, and often these are opportunities to change ourselves. Hands-on navigation—in the midst of transformation—is essential for your dependable and timely arrival. But here's the thing: True North is hard to follow when you're sleep deprived, stressed out and unwell. When you're at the bottom of your own list of priorities, you will eventually notice the negative effects it has on your eating habits, stress and energy levels, and overall motivation.

"I've never seen any life transformation that didn't begin with the person in question finally getting tired of their own bullshit."
– Elizabeth Gilbert, writer, biographer, memoirist and author of *Big Magic*

Every soul pilot loves the energy from a tailwind, but strong crosswinds upon arrival are another story. The influential forces around us are a factor in a large percentage of landing setbacks, and we need to constantly be vigilant of their direction and speed in relation to our destination. Our environment will blow us off course unless we correct for its effect.

So many of us choose to stay where we are even when uncomfortable and unwell. We sometimes prefer our unhealthy habits rather than facing the unknown. Too often we become so focused on other people and meeting their needs that we neglect to take care of ourselves. We take on too much. We don't get enough sleep. We fall short of prioritizing time for exercise or preparing healthy meals.

Self-care is the foundation for True North and the healthy choices you make in your life. Self-care provides insight and understanding so that you'll know what you need when you need it. When you become aware of how certain foods energize or deplete you, you'll be more likely to add or subtract those foods to or from your daily routine. When you're able to see how others are influencing you, encouraging you or otherwise, you can make conscious choices to connect with other soul pilots and create healthier relationships with those around you.

Most of us don't think of exercise as a spiritual practice, but you cannot create a rock-solid foundation for a healthy lifestyle if you don't give your body something as essential and nourishing as exercise.[23] When we exercise, we feel alive. It elevates our state of being. It strengthens our resolve. Strong bodies and strong minds go hand-in-hand. When you become physically strong, you remind yourself that you're capable of so much more than you used to be. Make your physical well-being a priority. Give your body some love. Follow what makes you feel well, and make your aircraft a vessel in which your authentic self can thrive.

"Crossing the starting line may be an act of courage, but crossing the finish line is an act of faith. Faith is what keeps us going when nothing else will. Faith is the emotion that will give you victory over your past, the demons in your soul, and all of those voices that tell you what you can and cannot do, and can and cannot be."
– John "The Penguin" Bingham, marathon runner and author

There will always be instances when following your regular routine feels impossible. Some days, you'll feel you're making forward-moving progress, while others will seem as if you're taking two steps backward. From a major heartbreak or loss of a loved one to a serious illness, accident or professional setback, sometimes the friendly skies can deliver some serious blows.

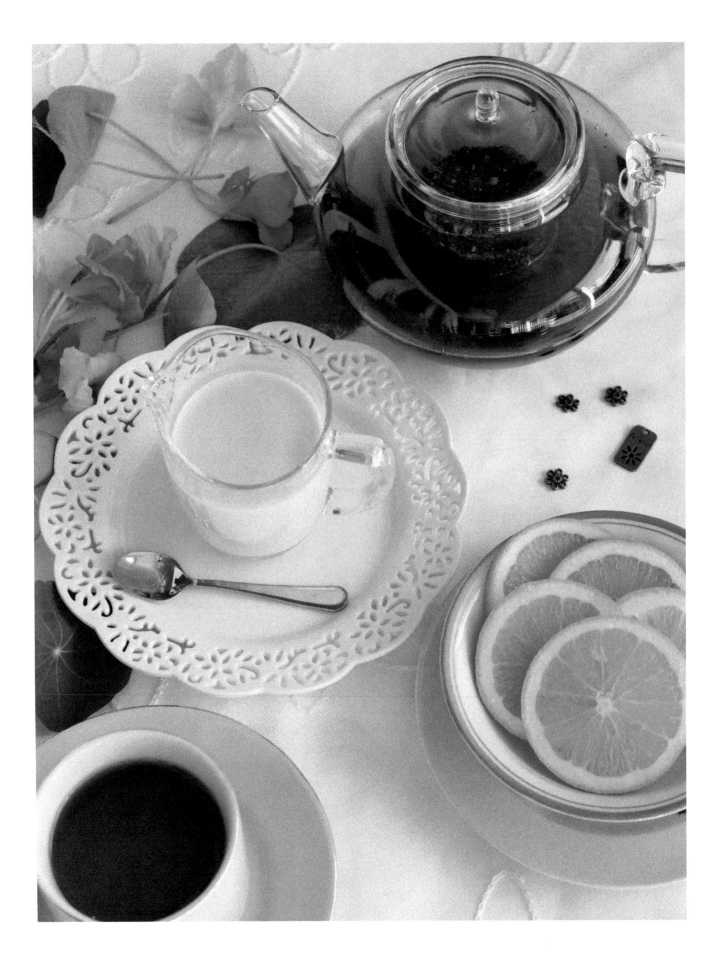

It's easy to drift off track, even with the best intentions. The most determined soul pilots slip up on their habits, too. What separates them isn't their willpower or motivation, it's their ability to course correct and get back on their authentic, true heading.

When we're not spending our time doing things that make us healthier, joyous and grounded in our truth, then we can quickly get swept up into the chaos of the world. And if your arrival is unexpectedly diverted due to forces beyond your control, you'll choose one of two responses: Resume when conditions are favorable, or start a new flight leg and rearrange to reach your destination by other means.

We are fickle beings with transient wants and desires. How we feel at any given time can determine the actions we will eventually take. For example, you may wake-up one morning and think, *"This is too hard."* If you attach to this idea, you might quit. But if you take a moment and reflect on why you're feeling this way, you may realize that it's because you have a tight work deadline, you're experiencing a health flare-up, your child is sick, or you're working the night shift (and pregnant). Give yourself a moment to reset so you won't act on that thought.

Self-care is your correction angle and direct track to your destination. It can be as basic as remembering to eat or as complicated as knowing and avoiding your triggers.

In this supersized, fast-paced, smartphone world of bigger, better, faster, more—it's important to step back, evaluate what is taking up unnecessary space in your life, and prioritize time to care for your body, mind and soul. **Each day invest at least 30 minutes in yourself.** What this will look like is up to you. Meditation for mental strength and clarity. A walk after dinner with a loved one for exercise and connection. Reading a book with a hot cup of tea for creativity and comfort. There are many different self-care practices and they're all easier to implement than you think.

The key is to find those you genuinely enjoy, and ones that fit with your lifestyle and values.

To embrace your True North is to never work against yourself. Opportunities for improvement never end. It's only when we take the next step that we see possible future steps. As a result, you'll fortify the internal compass that supports your continuous evolution. Your journey will always be a series of ups and downs. And when times are rough, a strong authentic core will get you through.

Any time you transcend limitation, you make a breakthrough. Celebrate and be grateful for each step along the way.

It may seem trivial to celebrate something as seemingly unimportant as packing a healthy lunch, but you're not necessarily celebrating the achievement itself; you're acknowledging and praising your habits. Your determined flight route can take at least three months to achieve, but micro-wins will happen on a weekly or daily basis. Celebrating your mini milestones gives you a reason to smile and dance while you're awaiting arrival.

You become stronger when you celebrate the small wins. It puts you in a growth mindset,[24] which allows you to leverage the power of progress and support the work itself. You feel pride and appreciation for what you've done and acknowledge the importance of the present moment. You remind yourself that you're on the right path.

Through in-depth analysis of diaries kept by knowledge workers, Harvard professor and psychologist Teresa Amabile discovered the **progress principle**: Of all the things that can boost emotions, motivation and perceptions during your day, the single most important is making progress in meaningful work. And the more frequently people experience that sense of progress, the more likely they are to be creatively productive in the long run. Whether they are trying to solve a major scientific mystery or simply produce a high-quality product or service, everyday progress—even a small win—can make all the difference in how they feel and perform.[25]

Here's an example of the progress principle made visible: If you're motivated and happy at the end of the day, it's a good bet that you made progress toward a meaningful goal. If you're feeling weary, disengaged and joyless, a setback is most likely the cause.

Create time and space to celebrate each leg of your journey. Find a place in your home that you love and make it your own. I have an "altar" in front of a big window in my kitchen with a bird feeder and a special view that I love. It includes photos, a candle, a Willow Tree figurine of a mother and her children, rosary beads and a jar filled with all the lucky pennies I've found over the years. Each morning as I watch first light and have coffee, I say grateful prayers for all that I've done and all that I have, and plan my day. It's my sacred space to celebrate the small victories and simple pleasures that brought me to where I am today.

Celebration introduces feelings of joy and appreciation, which fuels your engine of inspired action. This in turn promotes more feelings of joy and appreciation, which makes you want to continue to work harder and put more time aside for yourself toward your goal.[26]

Be on the lookout for your little victories. Reflect on them. Build upon them. They are the backbone of your success.

"Alis grave nil." (Nothing is heavy to those who have wings.)
— Latin phrase

At that moment of action—when all your hard work starts to pay off—perhaps that little voice creeps in to stop you from moving forward. It creates doubt and you hesitate to question your decisions. Not only are you faced with a setback, but you now also feel incapable of getting through it.

Jet streams are wonderful when they push you towards your destination, however when flying against them, you must fight an equally powerful headwind. You know what to do, but can't seem to make yourself do it. How do you get out of your head, stop thinking about what you need to do, and do it?

Self-doubt often stems from the fear of uncertainty. If we don't know what's coming up on the horizon or what our next step will be, we feel uncertain—and uncertainty breeds fear, hesitation and resistance. As a result, we begin to doubt ourselves and default to the autopilot of our old habits and behaviors.

Think of your resistance like the wind currents along the edges of the jet stream. This air is choppy and turbulent as your high-speed desire meets your more slowly moving, almost stationary doubt and fear. Jet streams are constantly in motion. Your aircraft can fly in and out of the turbulence many times in a single trip. To avoid the discomfort of this sudden change, you'll need to commit to the decision to fly through the resistance to smoother conditions.

Just like turbulence, periods of resistance only last a few minutes. The key is to launch yourself through your resistance within the first few seconds before you hesitate and talk yourself out of taking that next step toward your goal. Turbulence is uncomfortable—but not dangerous. It is a totally safe inconvenience, and very much part of our daily lives. Doubt will always exist in one form or another. You can't avoid it and you can't suppress it. Instead, you must feel your doubt and work through it.

"When you understand the power of a 5-second decision, and you understand that you always have a choice to go from autopilot to decision maker, everything in your life will change."
– Mel Robbins, speaker, CNN contributor, author and creator of the *5 Second Rule*

There is a speed at which you decide whether or not your aircraft will take off. This decision speed is your intuition. It can be said that intuition is your "commit to fly" speed and is the calculated decision point at which takeoff must continue. When you reach this speed, count backwards from five. When you get to one, this is the next speed at which you pivot into action.

According to Mel Robbins, counting down "5-4-3-2-1" helps to facilitate our intuitive decision making. It is a form of metacognition, which is awareness and understanding of one's own thought processes. When you count backwards, you're taking deliberate action and interrupting habit loops and patterns of behavior. It's a starting ritual that requires you to focus.[27]

Most decisions happen instantly and are made when we're flying on autopilot.[28] Our authentic self is who we are when we consciously start following the little nudges and urges of intuition, and let go of all of the fear, self-doubt and judgments we've placed upon ourselves. We're all going to deal with setbacks, but we can overcome them if we view them as part of the bigger picture of life and commit to seeing them through from start to finish. Recognize setbacks as a sign something is *happening*.

Arrival is only the end of one segment of your journey and the beginning of something completely new. It is the gift of a new perspective and a deliberate process for you to expand and grow into the kind of person you've always known you are—with wellness and peace as top priorities. With each and every decision you make, you'll reinforce your self-direction, mastery and purpose as they become part of your being. You will broaden and polish the skills you need to thrive.

When you become aware of your core values, every decision you make is easier. It doesn't mean that you'll never experience turbulence again, but when you are in alignment with your soul, you will always be steered in the best possible direction toward True North.

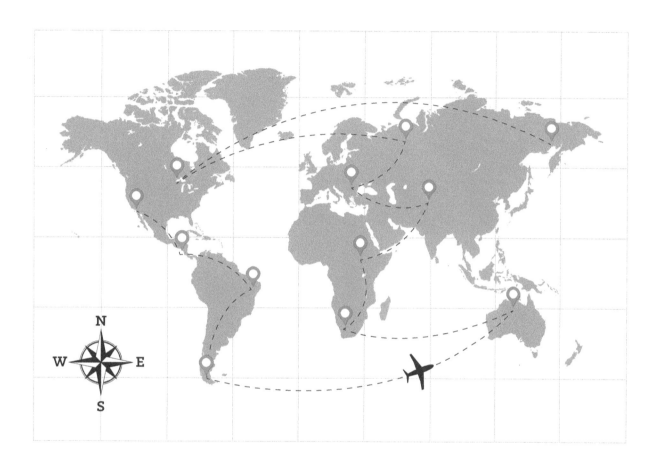

"Like a magnetized needle floating on a surface of oil, Resistance will unfailingly point to True North, meaning that calling or action it most wants to stop us from doing. We can use this. We can use it as a compass. We can navigate by Resistance, letting it guide us to that calling or action that we must follow before all others."
— Steven Pressfield, writer of historical fiction and non-fiction, and author of *The War of Art*

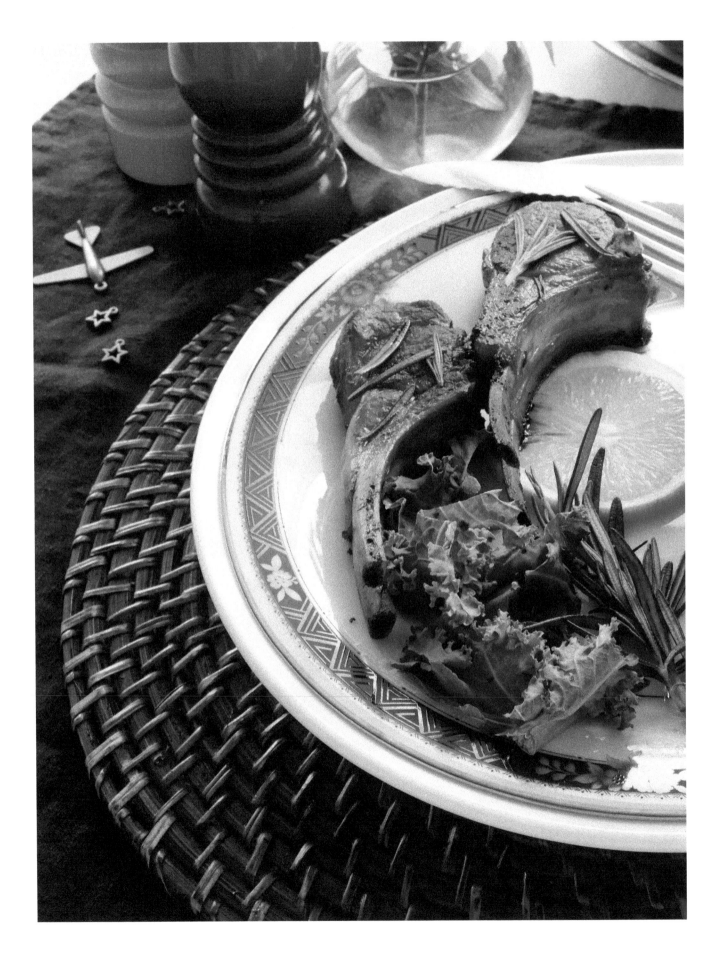

2

the four principles

*How do you move forward while
trying to keep your life in balance?*

When we're in an optimal state of dynamic
equilibrium, we naturally tend to listen to
our body with love and make choices that
support our health, healing and happiness.

When we reach our new wellness baseline, we adjust and embrace it with pride and grace. We're all familiar with the buzz that comes from achieving a new goal, however this new equilibrium also expects to adapt and change. Too much change at once can disrupt internal balance. Too little change can lead to stagnation. How do we adapt to our influences to help us establish the optimal state of dynamic equilibrium between our well-being and how we live our lives, so that it's natural and effortless to sustain that healthy, high flyin' feeling?

The first step is simply to pay attention to what is happening right now. Your life today is the sum of your habits. Everything is interconnected.

Just as you quickly adjust to the heat of a hot bath or a peculiar smell in your own home, so, too, do you adapt to changing life circumstances. This section features solid principles and proven practices to maintain optimal health and well-being using a holistic approach. It's divided into four parts based off of the four fundamental forces of flight:

1. **Knowledge** (Lift)
2. **Strength** (Weight)
3. **Wisdom** (Drag)
4. **Inspiration** (Thrust)

A force is a push or a pull that causes an object to undergo a change in speed, a change in direction or a change in shape. Movement in either direction means moving out of the known and into the unknown. We are constantly moving and adapting to the change around us, all while trying to keep the various elements of our lives in balance.

By regularly practicing a combination of the above principles, you will be able to maintain and enjoy a higher level of happiness when both positive and negative things happen in your life.[29] You are a holistic being, meaning there are physical, emotional, mental, social and spiritual aspects of yourself. Like the aerodynamics of flight, each aspect works in harmony with the others, complementing and enhancing each other.

Understanding how these forces work is essential for an optimal state of dynamic equilibrium.

A holistic system is a set of elements and parts actively interacting, organized for a goal. The forces acting on a system adjust as the conditions change, creating a stable system that can respond as needed when external forces disrupt it. A life in dynamic equilibrium has the flexibility to reorganize itself, evolve and adapt, all in the interest of conserving energy and resuming a steady state—a calm and peaceful mode of being that won't let you down.

Your health cannot be compartmentalized. Eating healthy, physical activity, a positive outlook, getting rest and working on inspiring, purposeful projects are all integral to each other for happiness and well-being. It's the balance of an organized whole that is perceived as more than the sum of its parts.

When you develop a harmonizing system for your body, mind and spirit, you return to an optimal state of dynamic equilibrium as a spirited, passionate and joyful soul. Your highest state of equilibrium is a combination that withstands environmental change and real-life circumstances to help you flourish as a whole. It has change, growth and flexibility built in, allowing for the inevitable ebbs and flows of life.

All of our life experiences point us in the direction to find and tweak just the right balance for our beautiful days on this planet. We only get one shot, so let's not tip the scale. We spend a lot of time trying to figure out the perfect combination of things that make us happy, but not enough time appreciating the joyful moments and life satisfaction we already have. Remember, it's a slow and steady integration of all four principles of knowledge, strength, wisdom and inspiration to maintain level flight. So, pull out your flight helmet and wear it like the high-octane pilot of your own personal Dreamliner. Let it mold to your spirit until it becomes a part of you.

Knowledge (Lift):

The foundation of well-being is the cultivation of our own self-awareness. This strong knowledge base and clarity of purpose gives us our lift. This can simply be translated as knowing what is good for you, what is important to you, and how you can do—and be—better. The more self-aware you are, the more you'll know what you need to get you closer to the things you want in life so that, on wings, you soar.

Self-knowledge and mindfulness are about understanding your own needs, desires, habits, thoughts and everything else that gives you liftoff to greater heights. The more you know about yourself, the better you are at adapting to changes that suit your needs. The further you pay attention to your emotions and how you work, the better you'll understand why you do the things you do. The more you know about your own habits, the easier it is to improve on those habits. And with a clear direction and a made-up mind, you'll have the clarity to accomplish your purpose and attract an authentic tribe that can support your being.

Strength (Weight)

Strength to be successful—reaching what we set out to do—has a lot to do with both our mental and physical strength, as well as the weight we carry both on our bodies and especially within our hearts. It's about creating the kind of life you want and being bold enough to live according to your personal values. Similar to our lives, an aircraft's weight will vary based on fuel consumption and the weight of its payload. This depends on the foods we eat, what we say "yes" to, how we manage our schedule, how many things we're responsible for, and if we're getting proper sleep and enough exercise. Sometimes, we need to take a load off to hit our goals and stay on the path we value. If it no longer serves you, let it go.

Mental strength is our ability to deal with increasing pressure in these challenging and turbulent times. It's synonymous with traits and qualities such as grit, persistence, resilience, emotional control and a positive attitude. No one has an unlimited supply of mental energy, so it's important to save it for self-care, meaningful work, building and maintaining important relationships, and learning. Your mind can be your best asset or your biggest weakness. Train it well, and you'll have the balance and stability you need to maintain a steady flight.

"God turns you from one feeling to another and teaches by means of opposites so that you will have two wings to fly, not one."
– Rumi, poet, scholar, theologian and Sufi mystic

Wisdom (Drag)

Wisdom is the capacity to balance that which is known and unknown with regard to experience, knowledge, and good judgment. Your personal engine, your healthy body, must experience drag in order to develop the wisdom necessary to cruise through life at the best altitude for your direction of flight. When we are in a time of adversity, we don't feel the growth that is happening in the moment. Only in hindsight, once we've found ourselves on higher ground, can we see how we've grown and the way we regard the world has now changed. By doing so, we free up a self-existing energy; the kind that enables us to work more efficiently and see more clearly.

Our ability to gain wisdom from adversity depends on how we choose to make meaning of the situation. When we push through the difficulties that can drag us down—consciously and without resistance—it frees our hearts and minds from fears and attachments and generates the full flow of our creative power for creating all of the wonderful things we want in life.

Inspiration (Thrust)

We can't accomplish our ambitions without inspiration. It is our personal propulsion system that gives us both the means and the motivation to rise above, be creative, grow closer to our goals, learn from others and achieve enhanced well-being. True inspiration gives a sense of independence and an ability to be autonomous and unique. It is the antidote for what drags us down and a powerful force behind our personal growth and purpose in life.

Inspiration is necessary for us to make progress and evolve. It ignites feelings of positivity. It pulls us from the challenging and impossible and propels us towards heights of joyful achievements. Inspiration can lead you to discovery by keeping the past aside. It encourages you to give more efforts apart from your routine. It endows you with the confident feeling that you are capable of more than you think.

Inspiration will wax and wane along anyone's journey, yet there are many ways to keep your engine of inspired action accelerating forward and upward. Inspiration comes from discovering who you are and what you most love doing. And the better you become at living an authentic life, the more your investment of time and effort prepares you for inspiration. You'll know when you're inspired as you start to enjoy the success from your efforts and the good feeling you get from them. It is from our own expertise in our lives that drives our capacity for further inspiration.

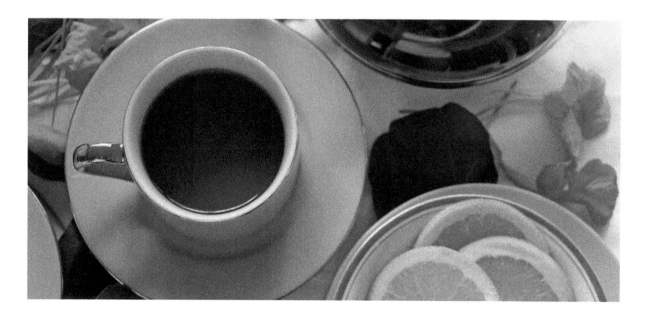

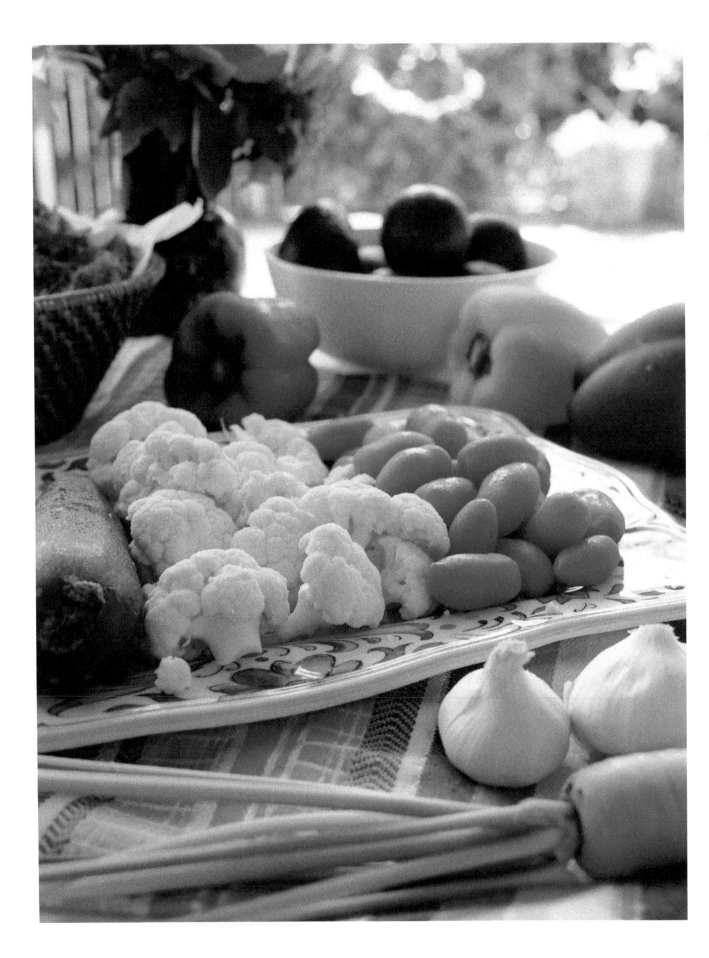

Knowledge: Lift

"Perhaps the most important force to a pilot is lift. Lift directly opposes the weight of the aircraft to keep it aloft. As the aircraft moves faster, lift increases until its force is equal to weight. When equilibrium between weight and lift is established, the aircraft is pushed upward. While lift is produced by every part of the aircraft, the wings create most of the lift used by the airplane."

Air in Motion: Aerodynamics and the Four Forces of Flight from Hartzell Propeller, Inc.

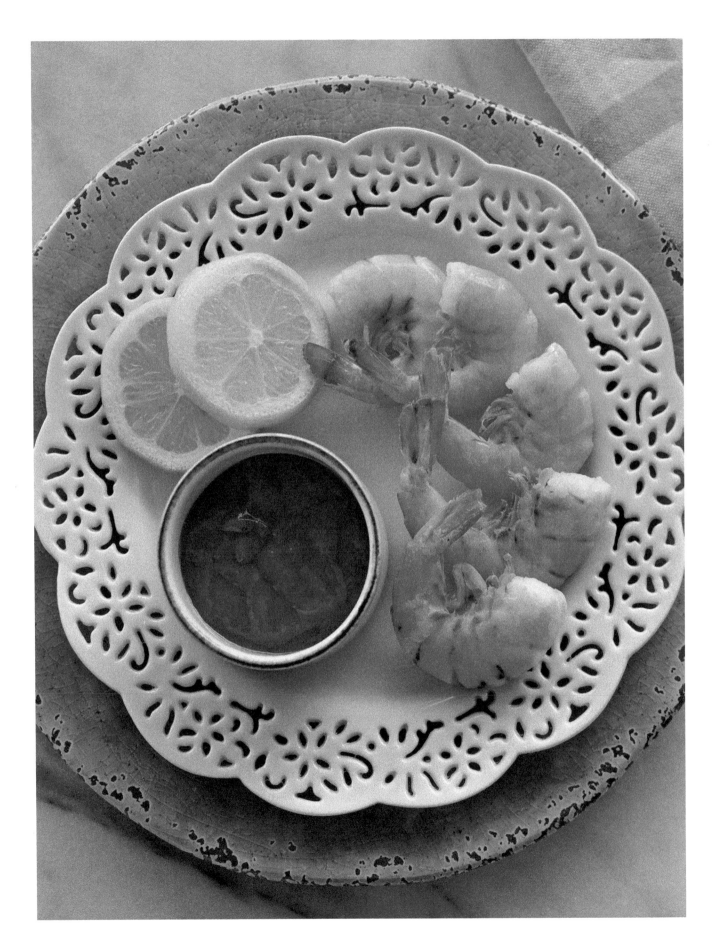

single-ingredient simplicity

The secret to eating healthy is simple: Single-ingredient meals.

I have found that the absolute best way to lead a healthful, gluten-free life is to eat the purest of pure things you can find. Whole foods that are more of a product of nature than a product of industry. The rewards are tremendous, whether you have a celiac or not.

Have you ever made a breakfast of a perfectly poached egg and a bowl of blueberries? Or, a lunch of a half-dozen boiled shrimp, a lemon wedge and an avocado? How about a dinner of pan-fried lamb chops in olive oil with a side of kale? If you shop carefully (or better yet, grow it in your own backyard), a single-ingredient meal can be so satisfying and easy, yet oft-overlooked.

When I was growing up in the '70s, and even still as I was raising my children, I unfortunately fell victim to food advertising and getting stuff to "grab and go". Looking back, I wish I knew then what I know so well now.

I was laser-focused on work (with my intense nursing schedule) and raising young children, so I wasn't paying as much attention to what was in my quick food choices as much as what I thought was the simplicity of it. Through my four years of college, there were the snack machines. It was easy to get a candy bar instead of a big navel orange or fresh grapes. A granola bar or a bagel was a full meal replacement back in those days. There were canned soups and boxed pasta meals, instead of access to fresh food. There were also the University and hospital cafeterias, and fast food was the right price. Not smart, but very convenient.

Consuming a diet of unprocessed, low-carb foods such as fresh meats, vegetables, nuts, eggs and fruits is the way to go. Really, for everyone. It is how we are supposed to live and what we need to do every day—not just some days—to be at our best.

It takes discipline not to fall into the trap of a quick meal or a sugar fix. However, once we do it enough, single-ingredient eating becomes so ingrained that we can't imagine living any other way. It makes portion control easy, too.

You may want to eat healthier, but the thought of preparing a salad with all the fixin's and carrying it around with you seems too cumbersome, so you grab something from the drive-thru yet again. But, how about a hard-boiled egg, a wedge of cheese and sliced bell peppers? Or, a perfectly-portioned carton of Greek yogurt with slivered almonds and a banana?

Any fruit or veggie, a fresh cut of grass-fed beef, nuts or organic eggs are all real foods with no additives or sugars and are truly what keep you strong, energized and healthy. A half-cup of almonds and an apple with a tablespoon of natural peanut butter will give you the fuel you need to hit your goals of the day. The key is to eat foods that start out as one whole ingredient.

It's really simple. For example, look at the label on a jar of peanut butter. If it reads, *"ingredients: peanuts, salt,"* go for it. But if it has a list of ingredients that you don't recognize as a whole food, such as *"fully hydrogenated vegetable oils (soybean and rapeseed), mono and diglycerides,"* then skip it.

Carbs get a negative rap because so many people are eating the bad ones. For folks without celiac, it's the refined carbohydrates in white bread, candy, cookies, sugary cereals and all sorts of other junk food and drinks. For those with gluten intolerance or celiac disease, it's the gluten-free replacement foods trying to imitate foods made with gluten that use too many processed ingredients and additives.

Whole grains are single-ingredient whole foods. As a whole food, they form a bundle of fiber, carbohydrate, vitamins and minerals. Packaged gluten-free products such as bread, frequently use only the carbohydrate component using refined flours from rice, corn or potato.

"Fiber-depleted, refined grains represent 85% of the grains consumed in the United States, and because refined grains contain 400% less fiber than do whole grains (by energy), they further dilute the total dietary fiber intake," writes Loren Cordain and Anthony Sebastian, authors of *Origins and Evolution of the Western Diet*.[30]

But, there are whole grains from single ingredients that are good for us. For example, popcorn. In its purest form—that is, plain air-popped kernels—popcorn is a healthy, whole grain, antioxidant-rich snack food. Just skip the microwavable kinds that use harmful chemicals in the nonstick lining of the bags. Instead, buy organic kernels and pop them the old-fashioned way on the stovetop. This way, you'll also avoid the troubling toppings that include gluten, fake food dyes and MSG.

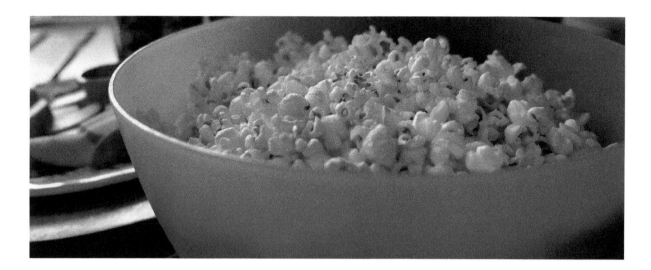

The supermarket is a place we go to feed and care for our families. We are the nutritionists, cooks, chefs, sous chefs, choppers, tasters, analyzers and final decision makers. Some us don't even think about it. We've been doing it from our whole hearts for our whole lives. I did that and loved it. I lived for it. I very much *still* love it and live for it. Food is love. Family meals bring joy. But, here's where it gets really important: We are responsible for other people's bodies, not just our own.

We don't always step back and think about it that way while we're doing it, but it's the truth. Going to the market and getting high-quality, fresh, single-ingredient food items is imperative to our health and the wellness of our family.

It's crazy to think that processed and chemical-laden foods have come to replace the whole, natural ingredients that our bodies need to stay healthy; that over the years as real food fell into decline, so did our health. We can change this!

If you eat only whole foods, by definition, you remove the processing and the dangerous food additives. A carrot, a handful of spinach, chunks of frozen or fresh pineapple, an ear of corn, an egg—are all whole, unprocessed foods. There are no refined sugars or additives, and there's no gluten. You don't even have to think about it.

The main takeaway: A daily diet of the most natural, whole ingredients you can find—combined with exercise—will restore, balance and keep you high on life every dang delicious day. Keep at it and don't give up. Your health *and* your family's health depend on it.

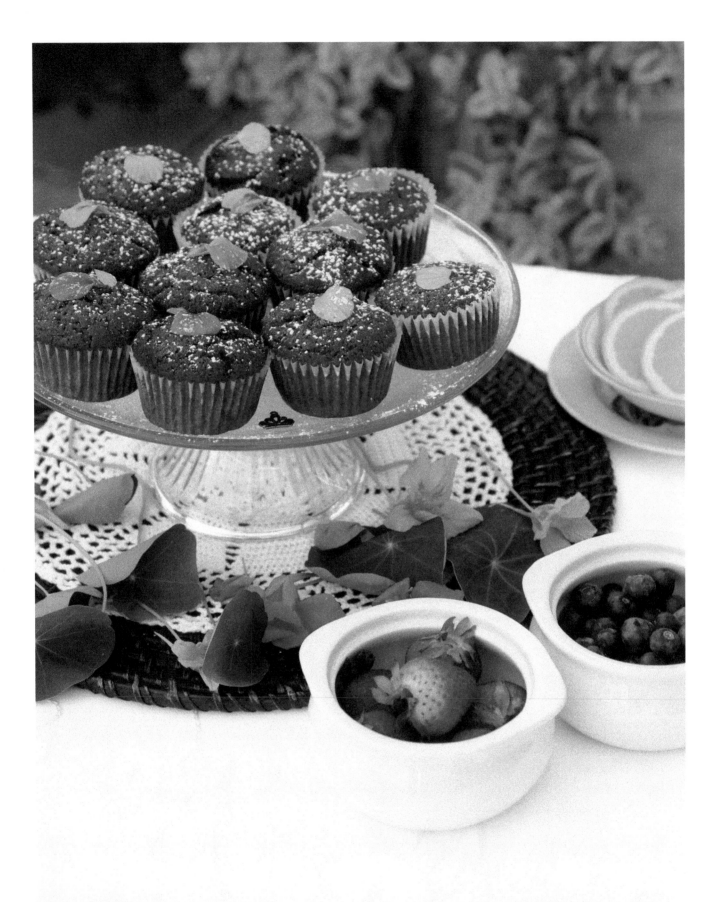

it's not magic, it's the 80/20 rule

You don't have to agree with magical thinking: Double rainbows, pennies from heaven... I'm cool with that. But, it adds to my day. It's a plus! I can tell you, though, that the things I remove—the minuses—are equally beneficial and keep me at my happiest and healthiest.

I didn't come up with the phrase "ditching the carbs," but it's a concept that certainly works for me. It's how I found an overwhelming positive in my gluten-free life. I ditched the carbs by following the **80/20 Rule**, or the **Pareto principle**. The Pareto principle (also known as the law of the vital few) is an economic concept that states that roughly 80 percent of results come from 20 percent of the effort.

We can apply this to almost any situation, including our health. However, when it comes to clean eating, you have to flip the 80/20 Rule and focus on that 80 percent. The breakdown as it applies to this is simple: 80 percent of the time you focus on eating clean, whole foods like vegetables, fruits and lean protein, and 20 percent is allowed for the occasional indulgence.

It's important to note that the 80/20 Rule is not a "diet" nor a "rule". It's a general guideline about balance and moderation to help you make simple adjustments toward healthier eating. Life is full of special occasions, nights out with friends, traveling to new places, amazing restaurants and delicious food. When you practice 80/20, you have the space to go out socially and enjoy eating the foods you love. And most importantly, it makes a healthy, gluten-free lifestyle feel more doable. Using this principle is one of the easiest ways to maintain a balanced mindset about eating healthy—without the guilt.

If you eat 21 meals per week (3 meals a day x 7 days a week), then 4 of those meals can be your 20% for carbs, gluten-free replacements, celebratory cocktails, dinner at your favorite Mexican restaurant, etc.

The day I sent the majority of those carbs on their way was the beautiful beginning of an energy-filled existence. Eating too many carbs is like driving with an empty tank. You're sputtering and running out of fuel. You just ate, but it can feel like the complete opposite. There are no reserves.

Even when I venture out of my routine (like trying the gluten-free English muffin from Denny's) it doesn't make me sick, but it doesn't do one positive thing for me, and I usually regret it. I'll try a gluten-free something once, but I want to feel the same every day. It's fun to introduce new foods and combinations to my diet, but now "new" has to include low carb or no carb. Fruits are carbs, but they don't have the negative effects that refined gluten-free breads and pastas do.

Refined gluten-free replacements are made from carbohydrates that are processed and transformed. Tapioca starch, rice flour, xanthan gum and white sugar are refined. You can find a lot of these ingredients in breakfast cereals, breads, buns, pizza dough, crackers, white rice, white pasta and pretzels. In addition to not containing any important nutrients, refined carbs can lead to weight gain, low energy and brain fog.

I find that the 80/20 ratio is easiest to stick with, but you can do 5/95 or 10/90 instead. Whatever works for you! The proof is in the pudding—and I'm stickin' with my plan.

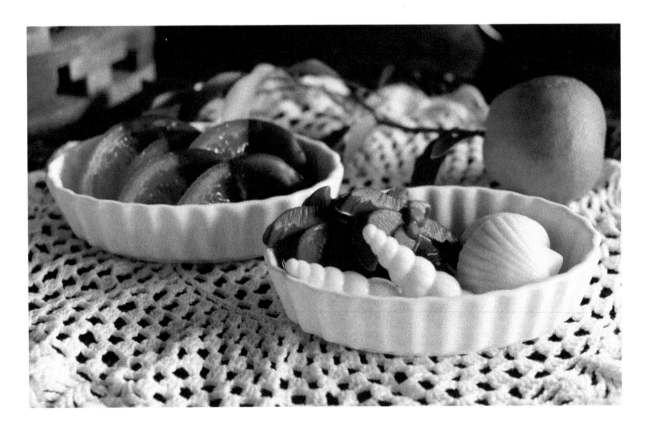

easy new year's resolution: water

Have you heard the Latin expression *sine qua non*? It can be translated as "without which, not". This may sound like gibberish, but it means "without (something), (something else) won't be possible". Water is a sine qua non for survival. It's the most refreshing and bountiful of all things.

We nourish our bodies, bathe, and wash our clothes and homes with water. We swim in oceans and pools for exercise and enjoyment. We sail, surf, wade and frolic. We need rain for our gardens and to hydrate the food we consume. It's necessary. It's restorative. It's delicious.

If you're like me, there's a good chance you think of ways to live healthier when another year rolls around. Most of us have exercise or food-related New Year's resolutions, but they're not always easy to implement. This can lead to frustration or eventually, not following through.

I've found that one of the easiest ways to do this is to simply drink more water.

According to the old rule of thumb, we're supposed to drink eight 8-oz. glasses of water a day, which equates to about two liters, or half a gallon. Some experts recommend even more. As with most things, this depends on the individual. Many factors (both internal and external) ultimately affect your need for water. You may also need to drink more water if you live in a hot climate, exercise often, are sick, or are pregnant or breastfeeding.

CNN Health reports that being adequately hydrated can help to ward off fatigue, keep hunger at bay and boost metabolism. "It keeps your body running efficiently, allowing it to work smarter, not harder."[31] I've consumed enough water within the year to attest to this. I upped my water intake in October of 2017 and had dramatic results. I love water, so this was easy for me. The secret is to carry it with you.

It began when I visited Atlanta to meet with Kristen Alden to film an interview. I noticed she carried a water bottle with her wherever we went. I also observed that she keeps a gallon jug of water in the back of her car. When she stops, she fills her water bottle. Efficient, effective and excellent in my book. I started doing this too, and have loved it. I unexpectedly lost weight and noticed a palpable difference in my energy level. I took this water resolution even further a few months later and replaced my evening cocktails with a Pellegrino on the rocks with a slice of citrus. I sleep better at night and wake up refreshed, which allows me to jumpstart my days and treasure my morning ritual. My skin looks better, too!

Consider this: If you replace every 150-calorie can of soda consumed daily with a glass of water, you save more than 1,000 calories per week, which translates to 15 pounds lost over a year.

I don't drink soda, but lost *additional* weight with my new mocktail habit, most likely from the metabolism boost and cutting these empty calories.

To make this simple resolution even easier, there are many foods that contain water. Everything we eat contains some water, and water-rich foods like vegetables, fruits and soups may help tackle both thirst and hunger. Raw fruits and vegetables have a lot. Watermelons and zucchini, for example, are more than 90 percent water by weight, according to the U.S. Department of Agriculture.[32] Different foods naturally contain different amounts of water, but it all adds up!

There's no magic formula for hydration. Everyone's needs vary depending on age, weight, physical activity, general health and even the climate in which you live.

Plus, not everyone loves water as much as I do. If you're of the camp that doesn't like the taste of water, perhaps you can try adding fruit or vegetable slices such as oranges, lemons or cucumber to boost flavor. Non-alcoholic drinks such as fresh veggie juices and caffeine-free tea contain mostly water, and all contribute to your hydration. Carbonated water is also an option.

A poem from my book *White Wild Indigo* is about this single-most important ingredient to life. It was inspired by a trip to Cuba where clean, potable water was not plentiful. I was witness to the country's lack of access to clean water and am incredibly grateful for modern plumbing, municipal water treatment and supply, water quality, and strong water pressure for showering. It made me stop and think of its importance, and not to be flippant about it.

As you begin another year (and perhaps a resolution), let thirst be your sine qua non to a more nourishing way to live. It may only be water, but without it, your good health is not possible.

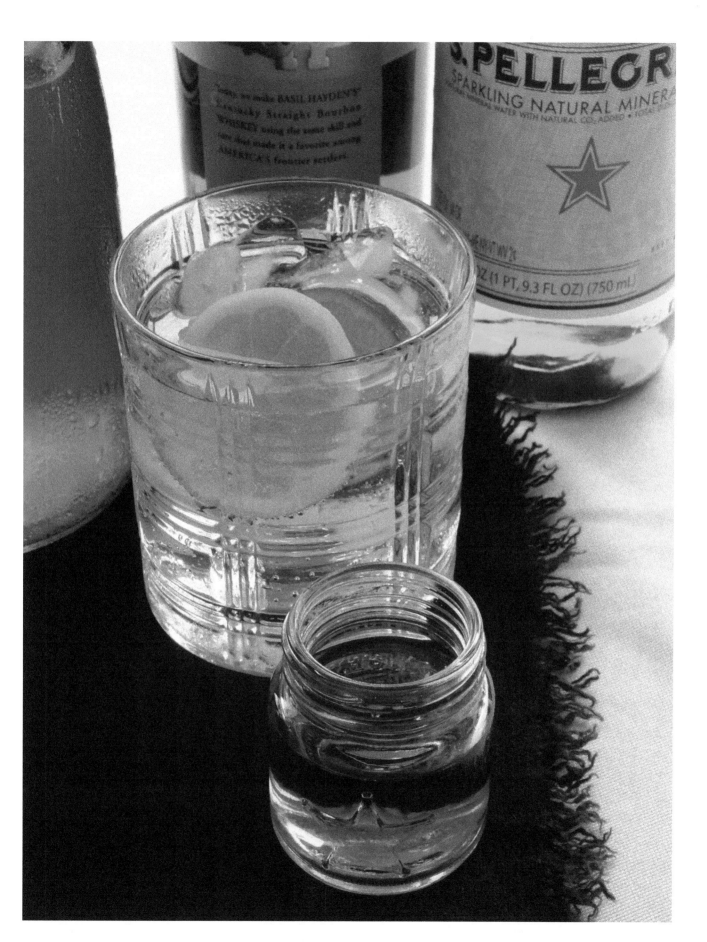

cooking with unconscious competence

Someone I met on a boat trip explained the Conscious Competence learning model to me, and then my son Doug mentioned it in an interview in the same week. This got me thinking about my personal experience with the gluten-free diet and what I've learned from my initial diagnosis to now.

The Conscious Competence theory helps us understand our thoughts and emotions during the sometimes-dispiriting learning process. It helps us stay motivated when times get tough; and it helps manage our expectations of success, so that we don't try to achieve too much, too soon.[33]

"When we learn new skills, we experience different emotions at different stages of the learning process. For instance, at the beginning, we may not appreciate how much we need to learn. Then, when we discover what we don't know about a subject, we may get disheartened, and we might even give up. This is why it helps to understand the emotions that you're likely to experience at each stage of the learning process, so that you can manage the emotional ups and downs that go along with learning a new skill." – From the *Conscious Competence Ladder* by MindTools

The Conscious Competence theory helps us do this. According to the model, we move through the following levels as we build our competence in a new skill:

1. **Unconscious incompetence:** We don't know that we don't have this skill, or that we need to learn it *(wrong intuition)*
2. **Conscious incompetence:** We know that we don't have this skill *(wrong analysis)*
3. **Conscious competence:** We know that we have this skill *(right analysis)*
4. **Unconscious competence:** We don't know that we have this skill, it just seems easy! *(right intuition)*

Pre-celiac I was a carb lover. No surprise, right? I loved corn muffins, toasted pound cake, and since I'm Italian, baked ziti, stuffed shells, manicotti… anything with pasta. I liked the pasta and ricotta dishes much more than the meatballs.

When it became imperative that I become gluten-free for life, it was a total shock. I remember roaming the aisles of the grocery store thinking, *"What do I get?"* I had no idea what I was doing. I made fried white rice. I tried the gluten-free pastas. I bought a bread maker and made gluten-free bread, but only after trying every gluten-free bread available on the market. None of them tasted good, and I felt like a truck had hit me when I ate them. I did this for many years until I learned through trial and error that processed carbohydrates don't make me feel the way I want to feel. I was absolutely unconsciously incompetent.

I figured out that a change had to be made, and that was when the conscious incompetence set in. I worked hard to learn, self-teach and focus on how to up my gluten-free game. I knew I had a deficit when it came to eating for celiac disease and the gluten-free lifestyle.

The better I became at preparing healthy, gluten-free meals, the more it became second nature to me. Over a 12-year period, I learned a better strategy and taught myself to intuitively cook gluten-free meals by working my way past the gluten-free replacement foods and into the outside aisles of the grocery store. I'm now able to cook without recipes and can put together a magical meal… entirely by instinct. It's become effortless.

Relying on recipes is one of the main reasons people struggle with cooking. It's why so many of us eat the pre-packaged, frozen and processed replacement foods. When you become unconsciously competent and can remove the burden of following a recipe, it frees you from all the stress, frustration and waste that comes from not having an intuitive sense in the kitchen.

Preparing all of your ingredients in advance so that everything is set-up and ready will help make cooking easier for you. Measuring and chopping everything beforehand also leaves you free to be mindful of subtle visual or texture cues, such as whether things are cooking faster than expected. For example, one of my recipes may say to 'cook until browned, about 10 minutes,' but that doesn't mean to cook for 10 minutes regardless of whether it browned more quickly. It depends on the day, the stove and the cookware. So, you must simply pay attention, trust yourself, and adapt as you go.

A meal is cooked with the mind, heart and hands of the cook, and instinct in the kitchen is not a destination, but a journey. It will take time to refine your skills until you reach a level of unconscious competence. And the more you make a routine out of it, the easier it becomes.

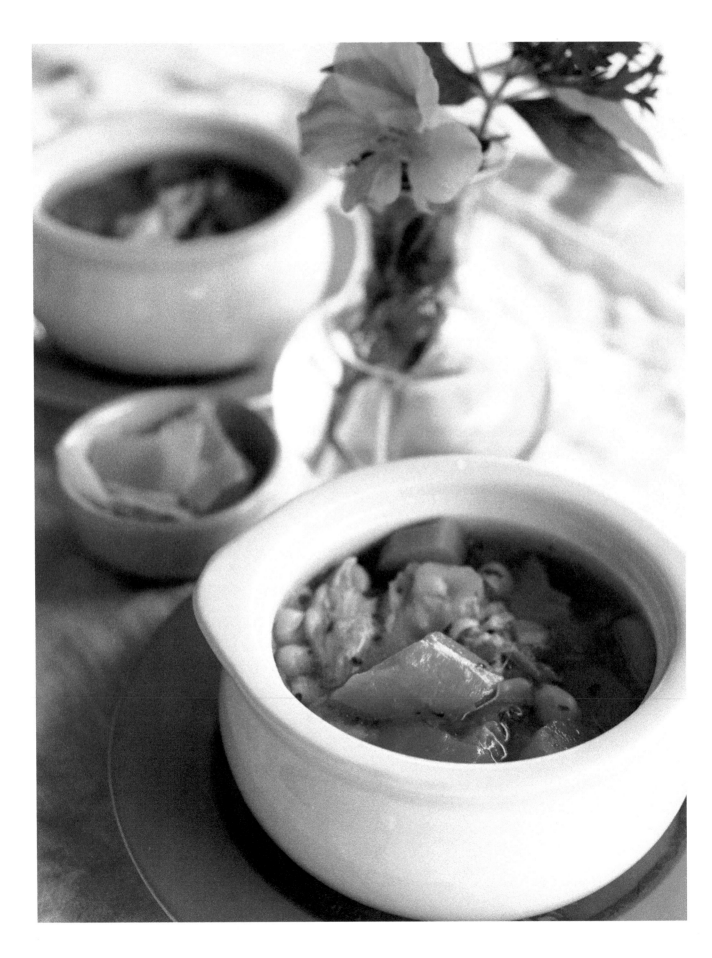

keep it stocked and simple

I like to follow the KISS rule for the kitchen: Keep It Stocked and Simple. The goal isn't to be the best cook, but instead to be smart, mindful and passionate in the kitchen—and really, in everything we do. I've learned that simplicity and smarts make for fantastic, easy and healthful meals.

The more I practice my enthusiasm for healthy cooking, the more creative I become. I'll take a risk on a new recipe, herb or spice. I'm developing my skill set in the kitchen at the same time that I'm enjoying the challenge of creating a new meal. If something doesn't turn out perfect, I'm cool with that. I tried something new and don't mind as long as it's testing my abilities and I'm improving every day with patience and understanding. My desire is to feel well and create meals from the heart. I'm happier when I stretch myself and try new recipes, and my family benefits, too.

I have three key things I take into consideration when planning the weekly family menu:

1. Healthy
2. Simple
3. Gluten-free

Well, make that four things, as I always add a dash of LOVE. It's immeasurable, fun, and the meal won't turn out right without the spice of life!

Everything I put on the table is carefully considered. Produce and meat always has to be fresh, or if frozen, be in whole-food form without additives or sauces. As much as I love to cook from scratch, I get busy or am not always not up for a big production and cleanup. Making my own salad dressing or grinding my own gluten-free bread crumbs just isn't a priority.

I like to stay stocked with single-ingredient, fresh, go-to items, and there's always vegetables in the fridge. I can wrap anything in a lettuce wrap or make a salad with yummy meats on top. I also keep frozen veggies on hand for an easy stir-fry or soup. I'm not a big pantry person because most processed foods made for the shelf are full of added salt, sugar and other unhealthy ingredients, but I do have certain things on hand for when I'm in the mood for quick n' easy. Amy's Kitchen has a great variety of gluten-free soups from which to choose. I also like black beans, nuts, and tuna for lean protein. And, frozen chicken breasts topped with Rao's marinara sauce from the pantry satisfies my craving for a home cooked meal without the fuss.

I tend to buy canned beans for the pantry, and individually packaged nuts, because the bulk bins can be risky for people who need to follow a gluten-free diet. Since customers often share scoops between the bins, you may be scooping your pecans with the same tool that someone else used for whole-wheat flour. Plus, we can't be completely sure that store workers properly clean out the bins used for one item before repurposing it for another .

I have a big bowl on my kitchen counter that I like to keep filled with bananas, avocados and apples. They are pretty to look at, easy to grab and go, and of course… gluten-free. A bag of fresh spinach and a couple heads of romaine lettuce work great for all sorts of combinations—from a spinach omelet to a lettuce wedge with a small steak. I keep two crates of 18 eggs in the fridge, always. This way, I can whip up a side of scrambles or serve an Egg Sandy to any hungry person any day of the week.

We all have those days when we can't make it to the market. Keeping your kitchen stocked with simple basics can help you avoid other temptations like fast food. For example, a bag of pre-cut broccoli slaw with frozen chicken thighs sautéed in a lil' olive oil and butter can take less time to make than a scoot through the drive-thru.

Carrot sticks and hummus will go a long way in terms of nutrients, fiber and feeling energized when you need an afternoon snack. A banana and a cup of coffee (no sugar) is a great healthful "fast food" alternative to any chai creme frappucino and biscuit. You certainly don't have to forgo these things altogether, but if you can stick to a healthful way of eating at least 80 percent of the time, you'll be able to see a big difference.

Plan ahead and keep your kitchen well stocked with your favorite single-ingredient foods, and it'll be easy to eat healthy when you're not up for the effort. Cut yourself some slack and let your creativity fly with whatever is on hand. There's no one to impress!

Gluten-free can turn into carefree once you master it. And, if you keep at it, you'll become commander of your kitchen, your health, the health of your family and lovin' life to the fullest.

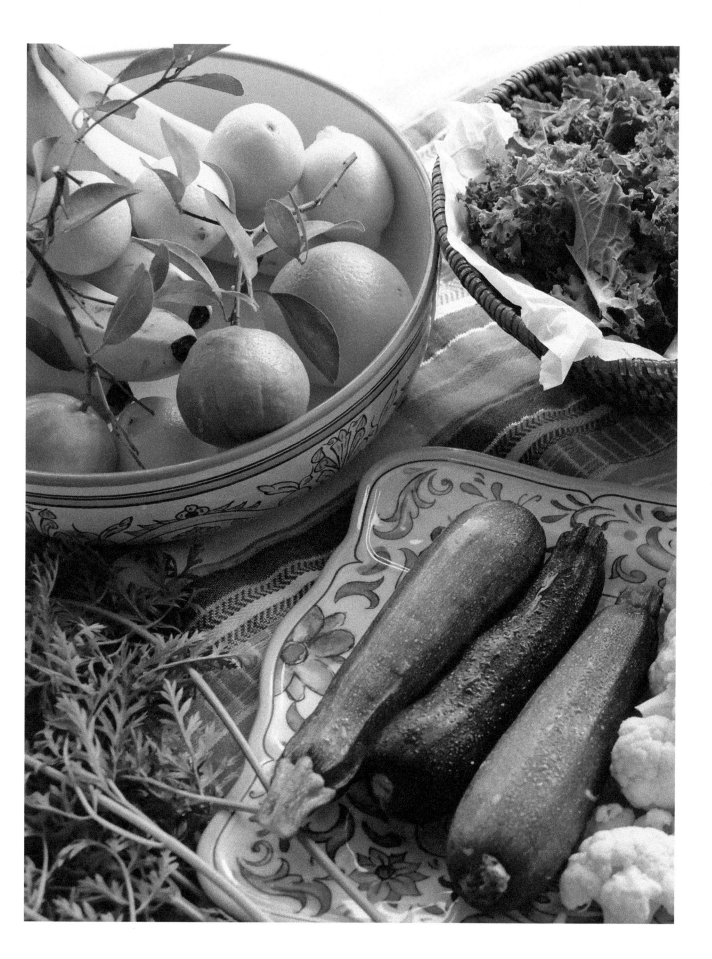

you're sweet enough already

Everyone has that one food that sends them off track. For me, it's the sweet comfort of fancy coffee drinks. I was never a Starbucks girl, but a former lover of Dunkin'… and at the time, I was flunkin'. To be completely straightforward, one of my blog readers suggested that I detail out my 30 pound weight gain from when I stopped eating gluten fourteen years ago. I often discuss how gluten-free replacement foods were a big factor, but there's something very important I haven't yet mentioned: sugar.

I was never really a sugar person and am not a soda drinker. I also prefer salty snacks over sweet. The exception was in adding sugar to my coffee in the morning and again in the afternoon. When I was first diagnosed with celiac disease, there wasn't much education around food choices and the gluten-free diet. I would order coffee instead of food when meeting friends out for brunch in fear of accidentally getting "glutened."

According to research, many frothy coffee drinks contain a sugar equivalent to three cans of Coca-Cola, or seven donuts.[34] These types of coffee drinks are loaded with other processed ingredients too, like high-fructose corn syrup, artificially flavored syrups and artificial food coloring. And, it's not just the frapp trap that'll getcha, either. It can be as seemingly benign as adding a tablespoon of sugar to your coffee. While that might not seem like much, it's so easy to double up in order to change the flavor from bold to sweet, or have more than one cup of coffee a day. It may seem pretty harmless, but let's do the math on this one:

1 tablespoon = 3 teaspoons x 3 times per day. A teaspoon of sugar is equal to 4 grams, so that equals 12 grams of sugar per cup. If you drink 3 cups a day, you're adding 36 grams of sugar to your day… for your coffee alone.

Sugar is nearly everywhere, and not only in frothy coffee drinks, sodas and desserts. It's in so many processed foods, many of which are the types of gluten-free replacement foods I've been talking so much about.

If you Google "gluten-free diet" the first five search results will give you a list of grains and starches that can be used as gluten-free replacements for flour. But, the majority of these flours

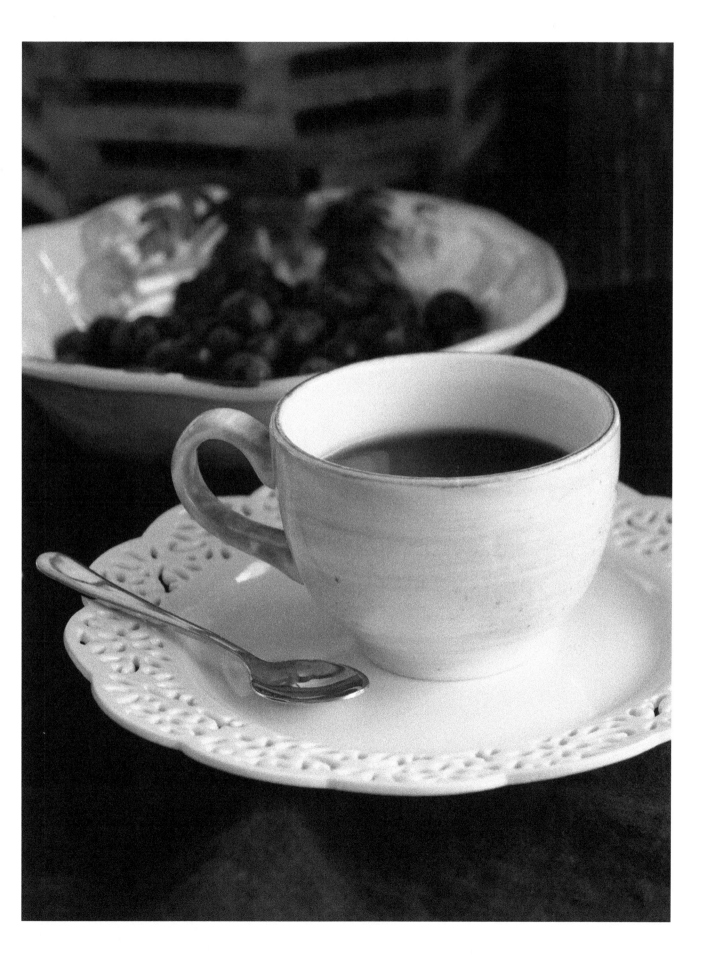

and starches used to make gluten-free bread and other gluten-free substitutes are incredibly high glycemic, which means that they can quickly elevate your blood sugar levels—and therefore your insulin levels—which lead to weight gain. In addition, when these gluten-free flours and starches are packaged for replacing traditional cereals, breads, crackers, crusts and pastas, even more sugar is added. Dr. William Davis calls these gluten-free foods "junk carbs."[35]

When you're gluten-free and can't eat much from the breakfast buffet, you might go for that extra cup of coffee or add some sugar in your coffee to replace the unavailability of healthy food items to get yourself going. This is a mistake. As tempting as this is, I can attest to avoiding that.

Sugar should replace nothing. Sweet comfort foods are not a substitute for bread. My thoughts are to avoid it altogether, though I know it's not as easy as it sounds. A study published in the *Neuroscience Letters* journal details the connection between food and feelings, and how when under stress, the body craves carbohydrates, which have chemical properties that soothe and relax us.[36] On top of that, add a celiac diagnosis and the emotions you experience after being told you have to change your entire diet around this disease. If the body craves carbs under stress, then we're craving the very thing we're told we can't eat. Yet, there's still the sweet comfort of sugar (and, we can so easily justify it because it's gluten-free).

It's important not to do anything that leaves you feeling bad. Too much of anything isn't a good thing. Trust me, I know this. It can be anything that makes us jump from the high dive without precision. Maybe the one thing that sends you off track is too much caffeine. Or, it may come in the disguise of a good thing such as too much exercise or volunteering.

Over the last 10 years, the three things of which I'm most aware—and that make me uneasy—are that sugar addiction is real, obesity has become an epidemic, and too much consumption of it causes problems. Many gluten-free websites are all about substitutions for cookies, cakes, and pies… with icing on everything. Take this for example: The Academy of Culinary Nutrition lists their recommendations for the "Top 50 Gluten-Free Blogs" with only few sites listed for healthy recipes like raw taco wraps, butternut squash pasta and roasted root vegetables. Scroll down, and you'll see that a majority of the photos include sugar-heavy cookies, pies, cakes and other sweet substitutions along with links to their respective gluten-free websites.

Just because you're thin and blood tests show no sign of diabetes doesn't mean that the amount of refined sugar you're eating isn't negatively affecting your health. Sugar is the new cigarette.

Think about the Easter basket you got as a child, or the plastic pumpkin filled with candy on Halloween. Kids can go overboard consuming the sweet stuff, and adults can oftentimes be children in a three-piece-suit.

The best advice I can share about refined sugar and junk carbs is that it's good to go pure. Eat whole, single-ingredient foods. Craving an afternoon cookie? Eat a banana or apple slices with peanut butter. Even a square of dark chocolate can be a good option. Yes, there are truly healthy forms of chocolate if you eat the right stuff.[37]

Most of the time when people start regulating their blood sugar by eating protein, unrefined carbs and good fat with every meal and snack—and, eat regularly (every 2 or 3 hours)—they find that they don't crave sugar and refined carbs, or even need as much coffee anymore. When you do this, you naturally have more energy and mental clarity, and are truly awake when you wake up in the morning. Listen to your body. Pay attention to cravings. Trust yourself. Much of what makes food comforting to us involves the set of experiences, memories and associations we have around eating it. It'll be much easier to have the willpower to say no to supersizing or skip the sodas and office donuts when you begin to recognize the why.

Omit refined sugar and junk carbs from your diet and teach your children this as a lifestyle, removing the choice. Reading labels is the key to finding out how much sugar is in your food. Look for ingredients like rice flour, brown rice flour, potato flour, cornstarch and tapioca starch. Learn to identify the many alternative names for sugar such as evaporated cane juice, sucrose, high-fructose corn syrup, corn syrup solids, dehydrated cane juice and corn sweetener.

The occasional, 20 percent of refined sugar and replacement carbs are fine as long as you have the tenacity to eat them in moderation. Everyone is different. For me, I had to quit cold turkey. I know all too well that going heavy on the junk carbs can happen in the blink of eye. Most break rooms, hospital lounges, or common areas in business offices have cookies, bagels, or a bowl of candy on the table to grab and go, too. The temptation is all around us. We always need to be awake to the presence of those Carb Dementors.

I'm so grateful that I ditched the frothy comfort-on-the-run five years ago. It has been an amazing transformation. I now get my sweetness in other healthy ways like poetry, my home or from the people I love. Everything in moderation—except compliments, kind words, or encouragement. Thoughtfulness in excess? I say, "YES!"

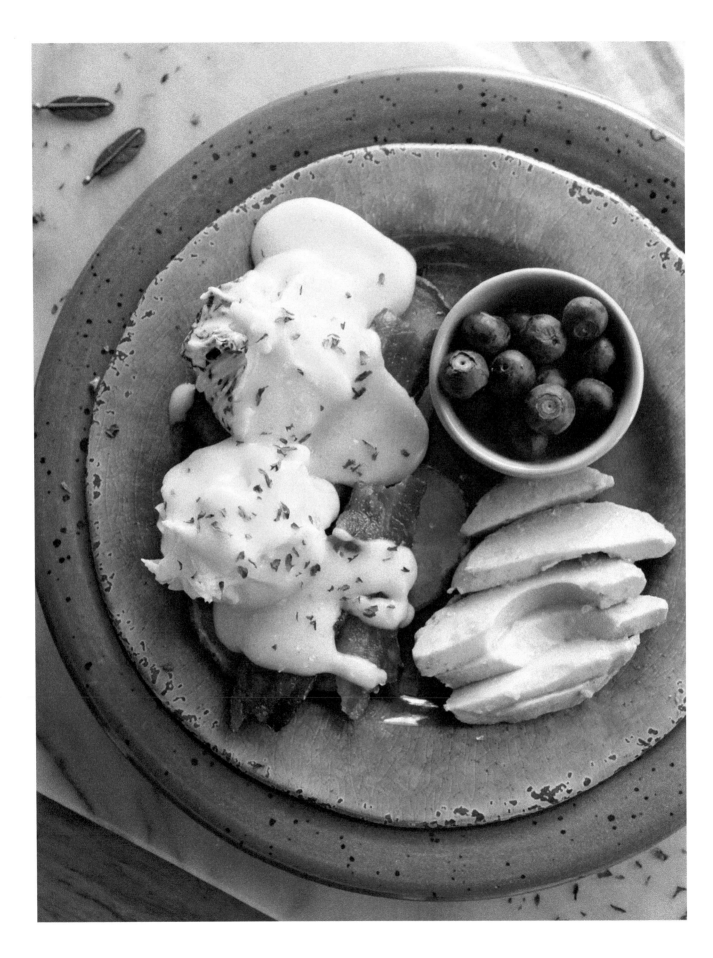

Strength: Weight

*"Weight is distributed throughout the airplane
and includes the mass of all the aircraft's parts,
fuel, passengers, baggage and/or freight. However,
the weight of an aircraft and its center of gravity
also constantly change as fuel is consumed during
flight. For this reason, pilots must frequently adjust
controls in flight to keep the aircraft balanced."*

*Air in Motion: Aerodynamics and the Four Forces of Flight
from Hartzell Propeller, Inc.*

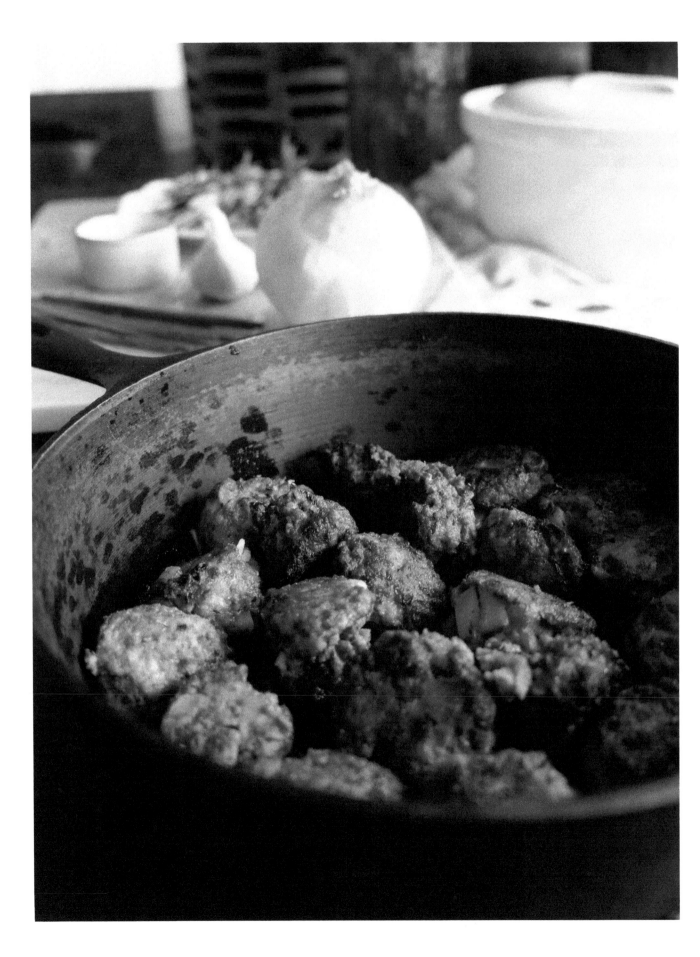

stay positive while going negative

Staying on a healthy track—meaning nutritious diet and regular exercise—takes serious focus and mental strength. You've got to be able to step outside your comfort zone, especially if your goal is to lose weight.

After many years of learning to navigate the gluten-free diet, I am incredibly grateful for rebounding from an unhealthy weight before my celiac diagnosis. I was underweight, malnourished and anemic. Any weight gain was a step in the right direction, and over the years I'd forgotten what a natural and vibrant weight looks like to ME. However, a good friend inspired me to think about that. Her words that caught my attention: "I need to take care of myself."

How often do we stop to consider what that actually means? We get busy; we eat at restaurants to save time. We want to celebrate a milestone; we call a friend to raise a glass at a happy hour. And if that happy hour is at my favorite Mexican restaurant, we chat it up over chips and salsa and the next thing I know, those chips are GONE.

I am not a dietician or a weight loss guru, however I do know that when you want to get back to your individual, optimal weight it takes some mental fortitude, taking stock of our eating habits, and goal setting. Habits are the things we do without thinking, and most of us are creatures of such habits. Take a minute to think of how many things you do out of routine in a typical day. Now ask yourself why. Do you do it because it is the easiest way of doing things? Or, is it because it's comfortable?

"Many people are skeptical about changing their diets because they have grown accustomed to eating or drinking the same foods, and there is a fear of the unknown or trying something new," says John Foreyt, PhD, director of the Baylor College of Medicine Behavioral Medicine Research Center. "Over time, habits become automatic, learned behaviors, and these are stronger than new habits you are trying to incorporate into your life," says Foreyt.[38]

But even when you want to change, old habits die hard. It becomes especially tricky if you travel a lot or dine out often. You have to squeeze it into a block of time in order to make your own food and control what goes into your meals. For example, restaurants slip in extra butter, oils, salt, sauces and toppings. If you're the one sprinkling cheese on your burger, then you know how much. It's hard to see exactly what you're getting when it arrives on a plate, already melted.

The first couple of days of portion size change and swapping processed meals or fast food for single-ingredient, energy-boosting ones begins with your creating space and time for it. It requires a conscious effort. If you're looking for long-term success, it can't be a flash-in-the-pan attempt. Changing your eating habits is an art form in its own right. Good habits equal productive behaviors, and breaking your own mold can only make you stronger and more confident to reach higher levels in many areas of your life.

I love to travel, dine out and discover new kinds of food, however these are the three things that work for me when it comes to keeping things simple so that I can stay on my health track:

1. **Prepare more meals at home—from scratch and with quality, fresh ingredients.**
   More meal planning and grocery preparation is needed, so set yourself up for success by directly planning what you are going to consume each day. Buy locally, in-season, and best-quality food whenever possible. When cooking from scratch, you know exactly what is going into your recipes. Non-processed, single-ingredient food choices can keep you healthy and help prevent weight gain, digestive troubles and allergic reactions. Cooking at home also allows you to control portion size and prevent overeating.

2. **Eat within two hours after exercising, especially in the morning.**
   Morning exercise tends to increase our energy for the rest of the day, and we burn more calories post-workout. It's also been shown that people who work out in the morning are overall more likely to be consistent with their workouts. One of the more common reasons is that when you exercise in the morning, you get your workout out of the way before the day gets away from you. When we have more to do, we're more likely to feel overwhelmed, and therefore, sabotage our efforts or self-talk our way out of exercising.

3. **Eat only when you're hungry, and until satisfied.**
   When you feel like eating, pause to ask yourself if you're hungry and why you want to eat. This helps you to become more mindful of your physical cues of hunger and satiety, and how you feel when you eat different types and amounts of food. It's a practice that strengthens our mind-body connection to help us understand what hunger truly feels like.

Forget the clock and listen to your body. Curb hunger by staying hydrated, eating slow and staying mindful of your bite sizes and portion sizes so that you're not completely famished by your next meal. Don't eat while distracted by other activities such as watching television, driving, or working.

To tell the difference between hunger and thirst, simply drink a cup of water. Wait a moment. If you feel satisfied, you'll know it's not hunger. You can also drink a glass of water before snacks and meals to keep hydration levels optimal and ward off deceiving hunger pangs that are really signs of thirst.

I don't weigh my food when it comes to meals, but do I follow a few guidelines for snacks. A handful of nuts is not what you think! Measure out a half-cup. Get some Ziplocks and portion it out. A small kitchen scale works, too. Read the serving size on the packaging. You'll be much better off than pouring those healthy, but caloric, nuts into a bowl and eating until they're gone. It's smarter. People tend to eat in handfuls when it comes to small, snacky things like popcorn or nuts. However, as silly as it sounds, it's better to eat one at a time. It slows things down.

In order to stay positive while going negative, you must remember that this is not a weight-focused approach, but one that prioritizes finding a balance between nourishment and eating for enjoyment. Our individual body weight is determined by so much more than 'calories consumed vs. calories burned,' like genetic, metabolic, physiological, cultural, social and behavioral factors. While your immediate goal may be to lose weight, this is about developing a greater awareness when it comes to eating, self-care and making more effective choices about your overall well-being.

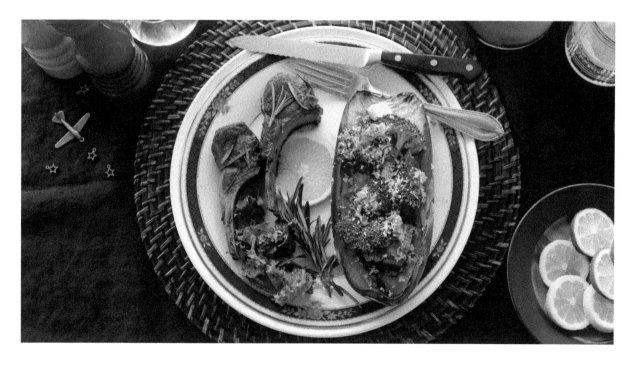

be your own personal trainer

It's best to learn this sooner than later to be a healthier, happier human being: Be your own personal trainer. Ultimately, the ball is in your court no matter how many gyms you join or trainers you hire.

You don't need a gym or a class to be in shape. You might enjoy the extra motivation benefits they provide, but it's not a necessity. My guess is most people feel like they don't have an alternative plan. They think that these avenues are their only choice.

You can be strong and in shape in your own home, apartment, yard, pool, neighborhood, parks... all around you. If you feel inhibited by the gym, turn on your playlist and dance in your own kitchen. Find a YouTube exercise video and follow along. The guilt that comes from paying for a gym membership or yoga classes and then not going weighs heavily on people's minds. And, once we feel guilty, we can get in a rut. We blame ourselves and this is not empowering. When we think that we've failed, we feel there's nothing else we can do. When we feel there's nothing else we can do, we often end up doing nothing.

There are times when a trainer is necessary to kick-start your routine. You may need to learn new skills to increase activity, work towards getting off of certain medications or recover from an injury. Or, it could be realizing that your inspiration is missing and finding a way back to it.

Your preference also depends on your personality and thinking styles. Do you need that external motivation and structure because you struggle with internal direction, or, are you the kind of person that self-motivates and is committed to your own ideas? Perhaps an exercise partner is the solution to give you the right amount of motivation and accountability to get you up and running.

It takes practice if you want to effortlessly carry a scuba tank on your back, cycle a 10K, or get to a healthy weight that feels good for your body. Establish a personal goal and a routine on your own terms. People look at celebrities and say, *"Well, if I had a private yoga instructor, I would look like her, too."* Nope, I'm not buyin' that one. We can't compare ourselves to others or it'll keep us from trying in the first place.

It's important to lead with *why* you choose to workout. You may have many different reasons, but the key is to identify the top three to four layers of why you want to make these changes. Keep asking until you uncover an emotion about something you desire or feel you're missing in life. For example:

Why do I choose to workout? Because I want to lose 20 lbs within the next few months. Why do I want to lose 20 lbs? Because my daughter is getting married, and I want to look good and feel fit by her wedding date. Why do I want to look good and feel fit? Because I feel confident and youthful when I'm in good shape. Why do I want to feel confident and youthful? Because I value fun, happiness and relationships, and know that I'll have more energy and interact more positively with family and friends if I am feeling confident and full of vigor.

When you love yourself, you want to fuel and nourish yourself well; you want to take extra care of YOU.

Remember: There's no place for guilt, blame or negative self-talk as part of the training. Look at exercise as something you are doing to benefit yourself. Identify the type of workouts you enjoy and choose something you love to get you moving. Concentrate on what you *can* do, not on what you *can't*. Replace all the reasons you haven't been active (knee pain, work, just had a baby, money, transportation) with a list of what you are realistically able to do. You'll be more successful as your own personal trainer if you're honest with yourself and align your activities with your personal core values.

If you're in forward motion, then you're halfway there. Keep it going. And every day, go a little farther. Be your own personal trainer and discover your true grit. True grit can be defined as someone's ability to persevere despite the presence of many challenges and obstacles to achieve a specific goal. It's the stickability that keeps you going when you feel there's little support or even negative feedback from others, or when you just plain couldn't make it up the hill as easily as you wished.

Express gratitude after every workout, and be proud of how far you've come and what you've accomplished. Gritty people tend to stick to their goals despite setbacks and perceived failures. It's moving forward with an attitude of "I can," and believing in yourself—that you can conquer ANYTHING if you put your mind and body to it—whatever the outcome. Put your energy into success. Believing you can has far more power.

your vibe attracts your tribe

My mom Annabelle, who is now 82 years old, was an only child who lost both of her parents at a fairly young age. She shows me what it takes to be tough, smart and kind, and to never give up. Yet, one of the most meaningful things she's taught me is that your vibe attracts your tribe.

I'm from a big, fun lovin' Italian family and was fortunate as a child to have a close-knit team of incredible woman who led the way for me. I also understand what it's like not to have this type of strong support. There was a time in my life when when my children were young and I was on my own a lot, *and* had undiagnosed celiac. It was during these years that I learned how it was ultimately up to me to turn my health and well-being around. It was also when standing on my own that I was reminded how human beings nourish each other (even more than pasta).

How does one person accomplish any one thing? What does it take, and what do you need to get there? There are three things that are—without a doubt—at the top of my list:

1. A rock-solid foundation
2. Mindfulness
3. Silent supporters, your tribe

Every day, you're building your own foundation, whether you realize it or not. Step by step. Brick by brick. With each action and every small, quiet step you take, you have the ability to create value for the world and produce work that matters, whatever it is you desire.

You're not just placing bricks to build a wall, you're building your own cathedral, or your own mini-empire, or your family or career. This foundation you're building can give you the rock-solid strength you need to handle the distractions and the unexpected. And when you're aware and mindful of this, it can become your superpower.

In fact, practicing mindfulness is one of the best things you can do for your well-being. It doesn't matter what you have or do; your life is no better than your relationship with your mind. When you can truly focus, then all your decisions, actions, and reactions can further enhance your life experience. This is a win-win! You are straight up paying attention, and the benefits are huge.

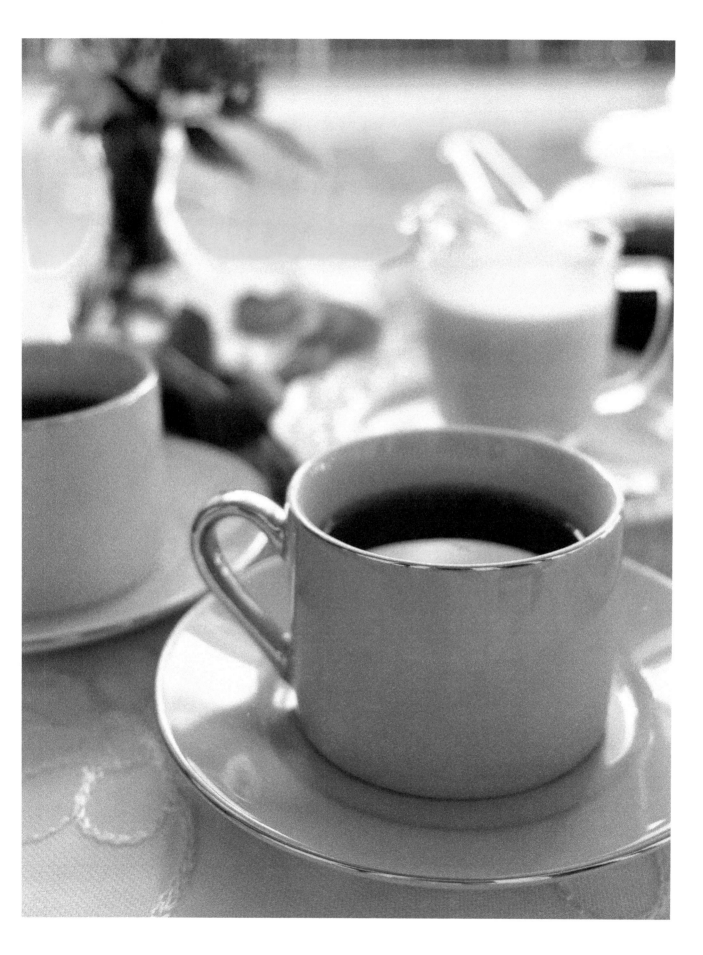

When we commit ourselves to the cultivation of mindfulness and gratitude in our daily life, we can experience life more fully and become truly happy, right now. Mindfulness also makes way for an authentic way to live. This is key when attracting your silent supporters—those who get you, who love you and will challenge you. Those who will not judge you and whose opinions you value.

Roy Baumeister, social psychologist at the University of Florida, states that "authenticity consists of being aware that you have choices and consciously choosing what you do."[39] So, when you exercise mindfulness in your interactions with yourself and others, you engage the authentic community that lights your fire. Your vibe attracts your tribe.

Momma Annabelle had friends everywhere, and I noticed their significance from a young age. They weren't "party at your house" friends. They were "Cheers" friends—where everyone knows your name. Momma Annabelle was her authentic self, 100 percent. Her kindness and reputation gave her at least twenty people she could call in a heartbeat, at any given time. It was fantastic to be around these meaningful connections and they were imprinted on my soul.

Part of our success is dependent solely on us as individuals, but part of that involves our fundamental need to be part of something bigger than ourselves. Finding your tribe is important. Acceptance, understanding and support are what we crave in friendship. With that heart-felt love and soul connection, we can't help but thrive.

I left home at 18 and moved four times before I got back to within three hours of Momma Annabelle's loveliness. When I look back, I sometimes don't know how I did it. Then, I'm reminded of my tribe. I watch what they do and remember how we all got to this point—that the energy we put out into the world is contagious. You get back what you give. This was taught to me by many and executed daily—practiced as a way of life.

If you haven't found a tribe, how can you attract one? What do you do? Like a magnet, you pull together your very own personal tribe by being brave, by being good to people, and by being your authentic self—whether at work, the post office, the grocery store, the dry cleaners, *anywhere*. This kind of energy is undeniable. It's my religion.

Show others the parts of yourself you may have previously hidden for fear of judgment. When

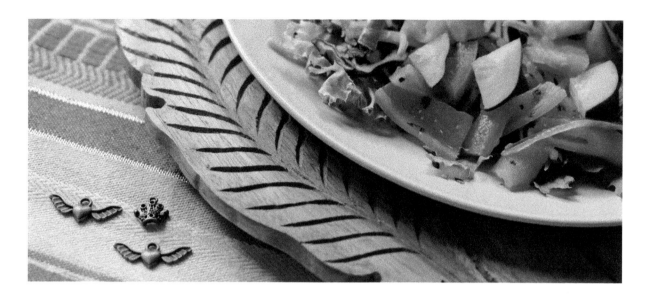

you're brave enough to show people your imperfections, they tend to do the same. And, as Brené Brown tells us in her fabulous TED Talk, *The Power of Vulnerability*, this breeds intimacy and fosters a sense of belonging, which will fan the flames of your soul's fire.

In early 2018, I took a trip out West and met many different people. Over and over again, I received the same message: Ethics, mindfulness, depth of friends and family, interests, goals, how you treat people—are all vital to living your best life. On the plane ride home, I read a book along this same theme, which inspired me to write about this. The book is *Asian Girl in a Southern World* by Dalena H. Benavente. It's a story of the author's life and how she never gave up with her stick-to-it-ness and courage. It's also a recipe book with some poems mixed in, so of course I loved it even more; a kindred spirit!

I keep Momma Annabelle's and my grandmother's strength with me. I encountered all kinds of situations along with my silent celiac. No matter what, their belief in me helped me to achieve many goals that, at times, seemed unreachable.

You have the ability to change or create anything in your life, starting now. Remember, every morning is a new day and opportunity to set your sights and energies on reaching your goals. It's ultimately up to you to take the necessary actions to help move you forward, but it's also a big, and sometimes insane, world. As Danielle LaPorte says, "Find your tribe. Love them hard." And, say thank you.

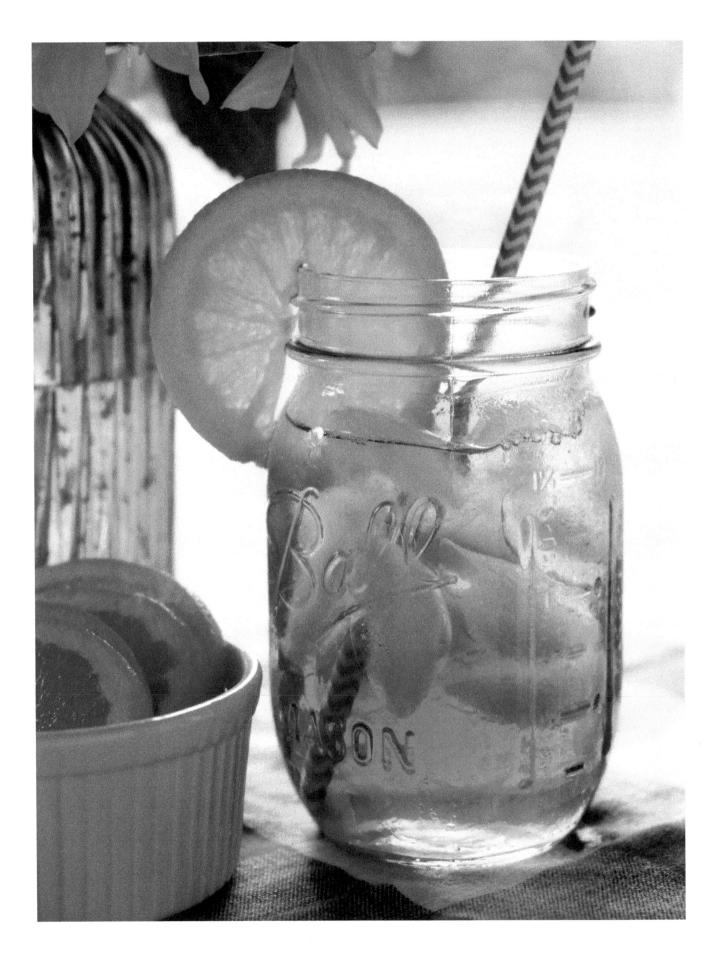

asset-based thinking

It's not unusual to want to skip a workout, or heck naw, not even want to get moving at all. Everyone has a bad day now and then. Even a bad week, month or year. We have to have a positive outlook, and most importantly, personal goals toward a bigger purpose to *keep at it*.

Positive thinking and positive vibes have gotten a bad rap somewhere along the line, but I'm not talking about some woo-woo form of enlightenment. Rather, they are ways of making a mindful effort toward authentic happiness backed by research and science.

Just think of what could be possible if we focus our attention on:

- Opportunities rather than problems
- Strengths more than weaknesses
- What can be done instead of what can't

This is the premise behind **asset-based thinking**. Asset-based thinking is a revolutionary, simple way of shifting our perception and thoughts to lead to positive change. The concept was developed by Dr. Kathy Cramer who says, "When you change the way you see things, the things you see change."[40]

Every day, we're bombarded with negative news of some sort. It's easy to become preoccupied with problems and focus on the wrong stuff. We need the right stuff—the things that lift us up and make our spirits soar! Negative thoughts are draining and dampen our enthusiasm and motivation. We can't have that if we want to reach our goals.

I'm a happy person and love life. I've also had my fair share of bad days. The pit we sometimes fall or get pushed into isn't going to stop me. I've worked damn hard to climb my way out. Right now, my body's strong, and I'm feeling well. I'm incredibly grateful for this, so I make a conscious decision to see things in a positive way.

But if you're feeling terrible, the term "positive thinking" can sound like a punch in the gut. So, how about asset-based thinking instead?

When you begin with a rock-solid foundation of positive thoughts (as opposed to negative), you increase your belief and activity towards a desired goal. Many people don't realize that positive thinking isn't only about the thoughts. It's also about taking action.

I understand that it's hard to find joy until you feel relief, but it's important not to let a setback mess up a well-planned goal and routine. The key is not to emphasize what's going wrong, but to come up with solutions for those specific problems—a healthy solution that's realistic and doable. A solution that can bring you the smallest amount of relief and joy in the moment. It's important to march onward for so many reasons. Feeling good is dependent on it.

So, what makes you tick? What kind of workouts get you inspired? What aspect of fitness and exercise intrigues you most? It might be Pilates, or running in the rain. You may have a wonderful gym or live near beautiful hiking trails, but simply need a push from someone to get there. I personally like working out alone, but have a buddy who keeps me accountable with regular check-ins.

Your home can easily be a gym with something as simple as creating a kick-asset-based playlist. Music does wonders for the spirit. Make a playlist that absolutely delights you. Choose favorites that get you motivated and moving. If you work at home, have your playlist going while you load the dishwasher or fold clothes—and take breaks from those mundane chores to dance! Maybe your kids will dance with you. If you have an office job, keep some free weights on your desk for an easy reminder.

You can start slow and do reps at different times throughout the day. I made sure to choose weights with an aesthetic that delight me, too. I love the colors and the way they feel in my hands. I use 5- and 10-lb weights, and do 22 reps of everything. Twenty-two is my lucky number, which adds to my joy. I had to work my way up to 22 reps, and now have a specific schedule to which I adhere. Workouts before, during or after work; a walk during lunch break; a 15-minute stretch session—whatever you can prioritize. Oh, and always carry water.

Some of my personal favorites to accompany me are: Archie Bell, Otis Redding, Rihanna, Dusty Springfield, Mumford and Sons, George Ezra, Tom Jones, Shawn Mendes and ZZ Top. Make your own special playlist. Name it something fun. Keep your list diverse for whatever mood you're in. Choose specific songs for warm-ups, and others to get your blood moving. *Hey Jude* by The Beatles is a great weights workout song because it's 7 minutes long—so don't stop until it's over. Play AC/DC's *She's Got Balls* and use your exercise ball. Make it so fun that you absolutely LOVE IT. The best part of listening to music while exercising is that it can make your workout feel easier or encourage you to work harder without feeling like you are.

When I first began swimming laps, I would use a lap counter and take photos of the numbers as they went up to text to a friend. This changed my life. I could exercise on my own with no judgment. Plus, knowing that I told someone kept me accountable to meet my goals. Some people don't need encouragement or support, but it can be like keeping chips in the pantry and trying not to eat them. That takes willpower—which is another goal, in and of itself.

Most of us underestimate the resources we have available all around us and can fail to tap into them. Asset-based thinking helps us reduce the odds of doing this, especially during the times when we need more support than usual. Look at yourself and the world through the eyes of what is working, what strengths are present and the different areas of your potential. Love yourself unconditionally—rather than only loving yourself *if* you do this.

Remember it's a marathon, not a sprint. Our instant-gratification culture has folks giving up too soon, and asset-based thinking is no quick fix. It seeks opportunities to convert setbacks into learning. These learning opportunities can then be used to achieve our long-term goals, which takes discipline. I worked on my assets and do exercise my way. Not feeling as fit and strong as knew I could be was messin' with my peace, and I sweetly and diligently said goodbye to that. We need discipline to go the distance.

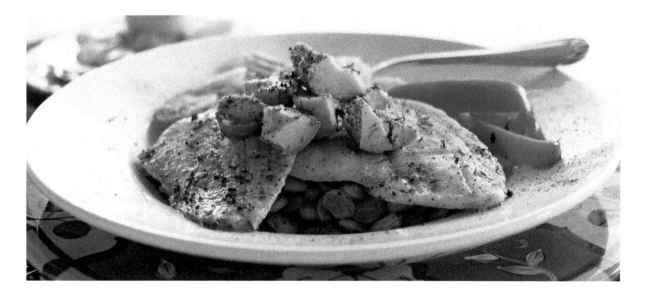

make your own 7-minute workout

I read an article in the *New York Times* titled "Can't Do the 7-Minute Workout? Neither Can I." It's a good article, but I was immediately put-off by the title. I wondered why.

It got under my skin because I feel it gives the message that it is okay if you can't do a 7-minute workout. With our 6-second attention span, folks might read the title and miss the very important subheading beneath it: **'How to make it work for you.'** Without that, a reader could possibly conclude, *"If the New York Times writer can't do it, then I'm not even going to try."* But, the key to success is you have to try. You have to get started.

We know all too well how tricky it can be to overcome inertia and take the first step toward change in any area of life. Any labor of love that's worth it requires stick-to-it-ness. Grit is the one ingredient you'll always need for the journey and it can take you further than any other quality alone.

I personally think that the original 7-Minute Workout is genius, but understand that it can be difficult. According to the article, the goal of the 7-Minute Workout is to exercise four areas of the body—cardio, lower body, upper body and core—in that order and as hard as you can for just 30 seconds, followed by five seconds of rest. This workout is designed to give you the maximum health benefit in the shortest possible time.

In seven minutes, each of the four muscle groups gets to work out three times. The key is to stick to the sequence so that each muscle group has nearly two minutes to rest before being challenged again. You have to understand this thinking behind the workout in order to modify it to fit your own body's strengths and limits.

So, how do you start on a 7-minute workout when you've putting it off because it's too hard? You make it easier. It doesn't have to be one of the thirty 7-minute workout apps on the market, or the one in the *New York Times* article, or a trip to the gym. You can be your own personal trainer, becoming stronger and getting in shape in your own home, apartment, yard, pool, neighborhood or park—and doing something that you enjoy and keeps you motivated and on track.

If all you do to start is march in place and stretch for seven minutes, you are better than you were yesterday. Even if you walk your dog for a full seven minutes, or move your booty while enjoying two to three songs from your playlist (approximately 7 minutes), there will be improvements to your body and well-being each day.

Begin by creating a plan that includes attainable steps around the type of exercise goals you have. For example, do you want to increase strength or overall physical fitness? Is your goal weight loss or disease prevention? Or, perhaps it's a combination of things. Start small and commit to doing 7 minutes of walking for exercise three days this week. This will help you establish new behaviors and create the habits you want to have in place to keep at it.

Here are the four different types of exercise and how they benefit the body, as well as examples of activities you can do to get started:

1. **Aerobic:** Improves the fitness of the heart and lungs. Examples include walking, swimming, tennis, biking, running and dancing.
2. **Strength building:** Increases muscle power and strength. Examples include lifting weights, climbing stairs, hiking, push-ups, sit-ups, and heavy gardening, such as digging or shoveling.
3. **Balance or stability:** Strengthens muscles and improves body coordination. Examples include core-strengthening exercises such as planks, hip raises, Pilates and tai chi.
4. **Flexibility:** Aides muscle recovery, maintains range of motion, and prevents injuries. Examples include yoga or individual muscle-stretch movements.

Fitness and strength WILL happen over time, and you'll begin to see health benefits such as the ability to walk up stairs without getting winded. Remember to eat right, as what we put in our bodies is the beginning of increasing our energy so that we *can* exercise for 7 minutes.

Working exercise into your routine takes a lot of determination and sticking to it long-term requires discipline. It's important not to set unrealistic expectations for a 7-minute workout. Seven minutes of exercise per day isn't a magical elixir that will completely transform your body, but it can be a great way to get your heart pumping and burn calories throughout the day when your schedule is full and you're pressed for time.

7 minutes a day... you can do that! Your body responds very positively and quickly to even small amounts of exercise.[41] Focus on beginning with just one thing and make it your own. Do you remember the workouts we did during PE in elementary school? Yup. We all did arm circles. But, the best 7-minute workouts are the ones we'll actually do.

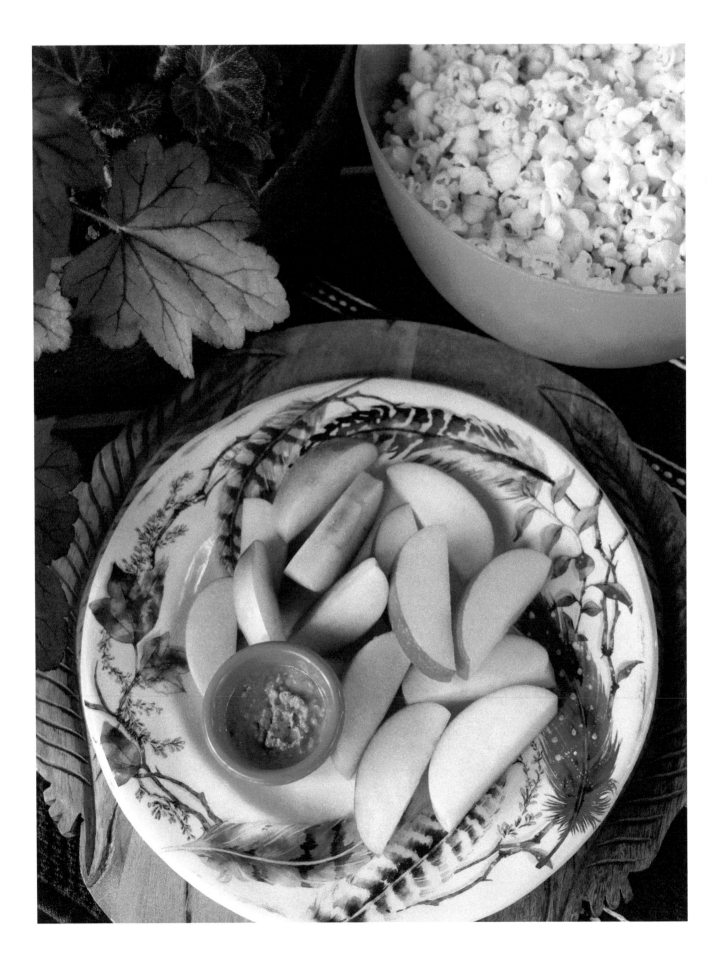

Wisdom: Drag

"Drag is the aerodynamic force that opposes the motion of the airplane through the air. Drag is caused by both friction and the generation of lift. Many factors affect the magnitude of drag, including the aircraft's size and shape, velocity, and the properties of the air flowing past the aircraft. Pilots have some amount of control over the force of drag by changing speed or streamlining the aircraft's body design."

Air in Motion: Aerodynamics and the Four Forces of Flight
from Hartzell Propeller, Inc.

rock-solid (and fragile) foundation

Have you ever heard the parable of the three bricklayers? I hadn't, until recently:

A man came upon a construction site where three people were working. He asked the first, "What are you doing?" and the man replied: "I am laying bricks." He asked the second, "What are you doing?" and the man replied: "I am building a wall." As he approached the third, he heard him humming a tune as he worked, and asked, "What are you doing?" The man stood and smiled and replied with a gleam in his eye, "I am building a cathedral."

A couple of years ago, I decided to produce a series of animated excerpts from my poetry book *Sage Words*. When I showed one to a friend, they were thrown off guard and asked surprisingly why didn't I do this sooner? I answered as gracefully as I knew how, saying that I was working on other palettes: assisting the artistic growth of my children so they could create their futures, working on restoration projects for our home and, more importantly, a successful family. I've thought a lot about that question.

To many people—on the surface—I was a bricklayer. Just a nurse. Just a stay-at-home mom. Quiet roles. However, I've been engaged and working with purpose toward the bigger picture for a long time, with each and every brick a necessary part of building something significant— carefully and vigilantly connecting the walls of my life, and that of my family. It occurred to me after this conversation that I've been building my cathedral. A rock-solid foundation has always been my goal. My loyalty to the project was endless. It's completion—monumental.

What can the architect accomplish without the bricklayers? The hospitals without the nurses and the families without someone to keep the machine well-oiled and running smoothly? We have to remind ourselves that the daily quiet, small steps we're taking are creating something of value to the world. We're producing work that MATTERS.

Why is it important for us to view ourselves and our work as significant? For when we view ourselves and our work as important, we also understand our purpose—and the significant cost for not getting our work done. The stakes are too high to stand still.

Six months before he was assassinated, Dr. Martin Luther King, Jr. spoke to a group of students

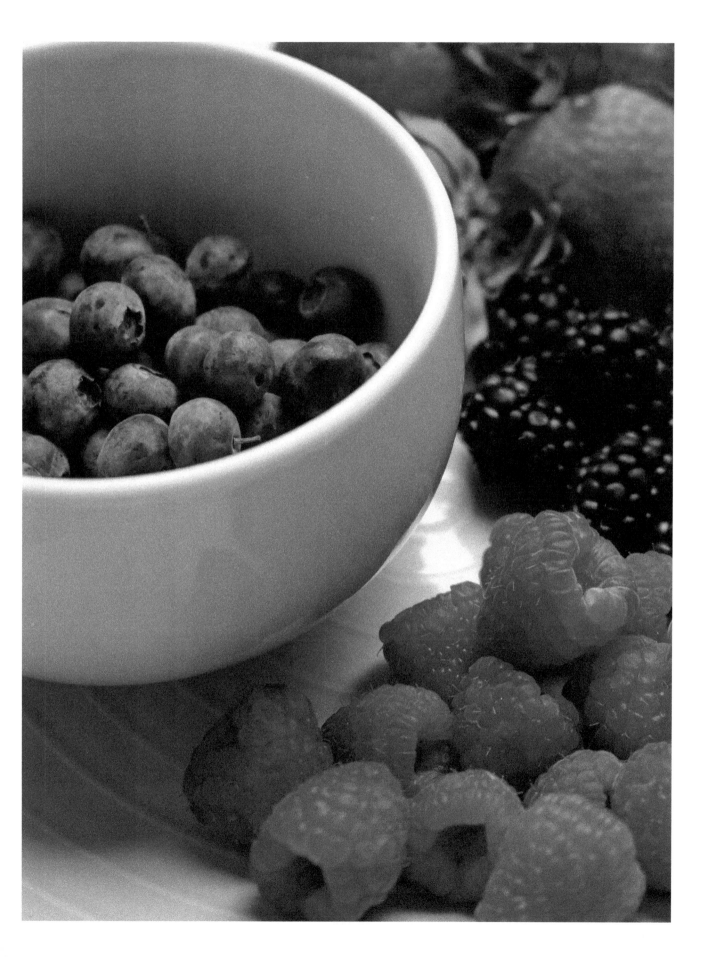

at Barratt Junior High School in Philadelphia. His question to the students: "What is your life's blueprint?" His speech that day—and this question—are a beautiful and poignant reminder that we need to have a proper and solid blueprint when building the structure of our lives. When we do, our lives will have ultimate significance.[42]

"If it falls your lot to be a street sweeper, sweep streets like Michelangelo painted pictures, sweep streets like Beethoven composed music… No work is insignificant. All labor that uplifts humanity has dignity and importance and should be undertaken with painstaking excellence."
– Dr. Martin Luther King, Jr.

The story of the three bricklayers is a tale of two attitudes. It was the best of times, it was the worst of times. If your attitude is positive, you can face life's challenges with a firm belief and a proactive perspective. Your perspective can determine whether you view your problems with desperation and despair—or whether you confront your challenges with courage, perseverance and resilience.

There are distractions and the unexpected that are not a part of our blueprint. Masonry buildings are brittle structures and one of the most vulnerable when under a strong shaking. It takes great effort not to get swept away in the earthquake and buried under the rubble. Throw an illness (like celiac disease) or a serious accident into our life's master plan, and now we've got to pay attention to our fragility. We don't feel so rock-solid all of a sudden, which can momentarily consume us.

But, that's why we build the foundation with passion and purpose so that there's solid strength to handle it. Challenging times can fortify our faith, strengthen our character, and deepen our resolve. And, we need reinforcement.

As you age, you become wiser. Life isn't a competition, or a game. As soon as your blueprint turns into either, you remove the integrity to do good, work smart and hard, and to be rock-solid no matter what comes your way.

As we lay our bricks, let's do it like Michelango painted pictures and with painstaking excellence. Let's respect that all walls must be joined properly to the adjacent walls, so that the ones loaded in their weak direction can take advantage of the good lateral resistance offered by walls loaded in their strong direction. Walls also need to be tied to the roof and foundation to preserve their overall integrity.

It doesn't matter *when* you give your time and talents a place to give back. What matters is that there's respect for the process, for whatever good is your aim. There's no right or wrong. Challenges can become opportunities, and vulnerability makes way for a powerful and authentic way to live. Some of us are young virtuosos and others of us are old masters. Our pace is the pace.

Keep the balance as best you can with your feet firmly planted on the ground, say thank you and breathe. Small efforts go a long way when practiced regularly.

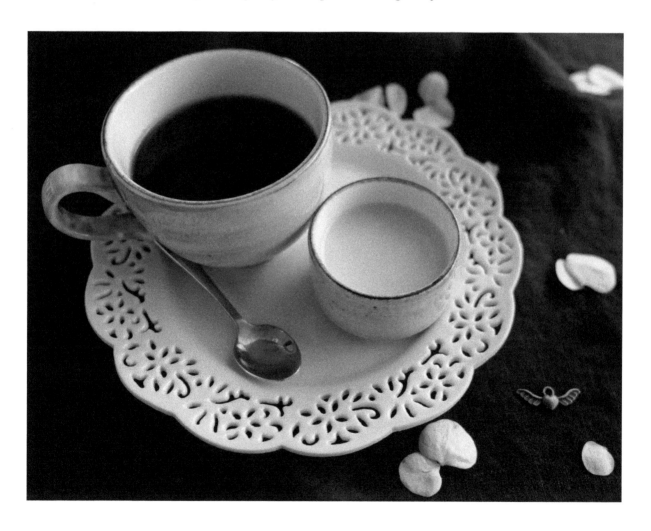

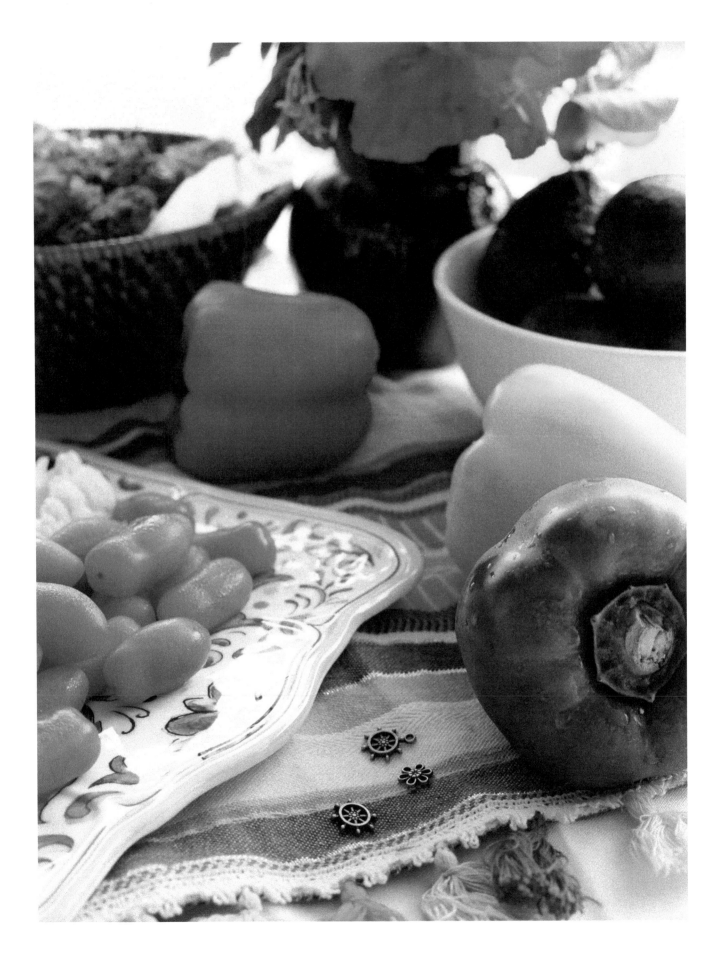

create the space for grace

There's a lot of negativity around the word 'workaholic.' I feel that it's often inaccurately used to describe someone who simply loves the work that they do and is dedicated to their big-picture vision. Can you be a healthy workaholic? Yes, but it requires **grace**.

I admit that I've been focused and ardent about my work. I'm proud of it. There is one *very* important thing that I learned from this, though. It's that our tunnel vision and discipline can be the thing that gets us high on life... or punches us in the gut.

You might be a workaholic with razor-sharp focus, but pay attention so that it doesn't become a detriment to another aspect of your life. For example, your posture while sitting at your desk, regularly skipping workouts, eating processed foods to save time, family conflict or emotional and physical exhaustion. Or, perhaps you are the workaholic who turns your drive and dedication into a healthy devotion to your business, goals, purpose, self-care and being mindful when someone has something to share with you.

Take care of yourself as you work your butt off to pay your bills and raise your children. Throw in an illness or accident, and you may have to narrow your focus a bit further until your kiddos get older. The ones who love you will know your attention is on their safety and well-being. They know this is the hat you're wearing for a while and will be patient.

There's nothing wrong with being engaged and dedicated to your work, and enjoying it immensely. Some of us have an internal drive that causes us to work hard and be more willing to make sacrifices in order to reach our goals. I loved parenting my two boys and can now look back with incredible pride as I watch them continue on to achieve and succeed. The gut punch comes when you lose perspective. Just as with everything else in life, moderation is vital when it comes to working toward the things that are important to you.

Think about this: Balance is a mix of work, wellness and creating. If you apply the focus and dedication you have for your work to your desire for equilibrium in all aspects of your life, you may be surprised at how easy it is to create a healthy, well-rounded lifestyle that centers on your happiness and the well-being of those around you.

To be a high-on-life, healthy workaholic, you must constantly remind yourself that work is not everything. Inspiration comes from life, and most of life's answers are hidden in the things all around us. When we slow down the pace, we give ourselves a space for grace that allows us to reflect, rejuvenate and restore. When we create this place and space, we have direct access to our deep wisdom and our authentic self. Why is this important? From this place arise the answers and solutions to life's challenges. From this space we begin to trust ourselves.

Way back when, I became a total blonde, though it didn't work for me (Ha, I'm Italian!). When I look back on photos from that time, I know now that I was exploring and experimenting. Sometimes an experiment works and sometimes it doesn't. The only way to see if it'll work is to try. You can't make, create, do or start anything worthwhile if you're not willing to experiment.

When you become bold enough to experiment (and, sometimes fall), you are putting yourself out there. And when you put yourself out there, people will have an opinion. This can either interfere with how you define your authentic self, or truly help you find your core being as long as you confidently know what those opinions mean to you.

In our quest to understand ourselves, grace is what reminds us that we are not alone, unguided or unsupported, when the solitude of our chosen paths can make us feel misunderstood.

A healthy workaholic needs proper perspective. When we stay in tunnel vision mode for too long, we pass by the finer points of life such as friends, family, children and even incredible, starry nights. Hard work should be balanced with sleep, nature, good books, wellness, healthy food and loving souls that warm your heart at the same time. Say grateful prayers each morning at first light, throughout the day and as you fall asleep. You can't work well on an empty fuel tank, and that includes your body and soul.

"You should always carry peace within you. It's the most beautifying thing you could ever have or do. Peace makes your heart beautiful and it makes you look beautiful, too. You want to have perfect physical posture when you stand, sit, and walk, and peace is the perfect posture of the soul. Peace creates grace—and grace gives peace."

– C. JoyBell C., poet, author and mentor

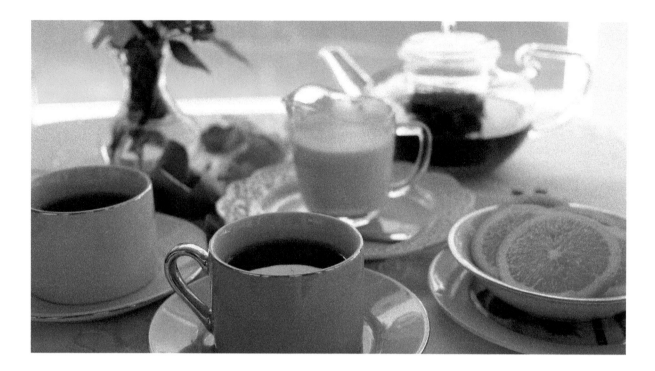

Grace is present in the beauty, love, kindness and compassion that is all around us. We can either create the space to notice it or take it for granted. You create a sacred space for grace when you choose peace over chaos and when you intend to live with acceptance, awareness and joy in each moment. Notice where grace seeks to connect with you. A good artist knows that it's the negative space that defines the object—the positive space—and brings balance to a composition. A good actor knows that the tension is the force that drives the drama, however, it's the most difficult element to understand because you cannot see or touch it.

As you let go of busyness, things may feel empty at first. This emptiness can feel painful or lonely. But in order to do the work we feel so passionate about and to maintain our health as we love and serve our families and communities, we must learn to create space for our souls to breathe. This means less *filling* space with work and more *creating* space where you can rest. Empty space; all for you. Feel into the present moment. Ask your soul where to place your next step.

I believe in working hard with passion and purpose, but also know from experience how important it is to take the time to regenerate and renew the best you can. Look up; it's free! See the birds and the stars. You'll miss the rainbow if you don't peek out after the rain.

where healing takes place

Some people are good at math and know it as well as their own skin. They memorize theories and can solve problems in seconds. If you open any math book, you can feel the writer's love of numbers, and it's as if they have their own language.

When I was younger, I had no idea of the vast degree of non-textbook math books available nor the extent to which these authors leisurely enjoyed numbers for sport. People who love numbers are just as prominent as people who love words, foreign languages and sports. Math doesn't get as much coverage.

Whatever it is that lights a fire inside you: poetry, science, math, music, wildlife, foreign language... it doesn't matter. My friend Jim worked at NASA for his entire career. When he retired, he became a hiking and bird expert. His enthusiasm is so contagious and inspiring. He hikes almost every day and takes amazing photos of interesting wildlife. He sends emails with attachments of a lovely creature that he's captured on film, along with an explanation of the experience. I always look forward to checking my inbox because I know something delightful will be there waiting for me. It's a beautiful thing.

The friends I have who play an instrument and share their music, or those who love cooking and share their recipes, are just as interesting to me because they're doing what they love. I was talking to my friend Jody about art. He's been playing piano since he was six years old and is the most fantastic, expressive pianist I've ever met. He's always had beautiful conditions in which to play and to be himself.

We briefly touched on how people are often worried about how they will pay for daycare, rent, mortgage or a car payment, and how they'll muster the energy or time to enjoy a hobby or creative pastime. Life gets busy and you've gotta make ends meet.

So many things go by the wayside when you're focused on keeping your kids, house, career or relationships afloat. Spending time on anything unnecessary to everyday survival is simply not practical. And if you've experienced a trauma such as a loss or an illness, how do you move past operating in survival mode and learn to embrace life again?

An often overlooked and incredibly important aspect of finding what ignites your soul's fire is the need to be well. It's not easy to explore, learn about or enjoy the world around you if you're not strong and healthy. Part of getting out of survival mode means having time to yourself. You need to create this in any way that you can.

The simplest way to do this is by taking care of your body. Eat well. Get plenty of sleep every night. Exercise every day. When your everday environment and your body's wellness align, it will become much easier for you to do what you love.

As my oldest son explained to me, he swam when he was younger because of the team aspect. He did it for the team and it was his sport. But when he started running, the gradual process of building on something made him feel better. Every day, he would add more distance, and therefore, gain strength and endurance. The more he ran, the more he loved it.

Swimming was to stay in shape. Running gave his life shape.

We don't plan for illness, injuries or stress. And when they catch us by surprise, they can dramatically change our lives. Commitment to exercise played a *big* part in my health and recovery after being diagnosed with celiac disease, as did writing poetry. I didn't realize it at the time, but while I was building muscle and physical strength, I was also building emotional fitness. I was using art as therapy. I was feeling hope and inspiration again. I was healing.

"Art is one resource that can lead us back to a more accurate assessment of what is valuable by working against habit and inviting us to recalibrate what we admire or love."
– from *Art As Therapy* by Alain de Botton and John Armstrong

The beauty of art—whether it be poetry, painting, dancing, music or mathematics—lies in the process. We enrich our lives by opening up the power of our imagination to discover our own wisdom and resilience through creative problem solving and self-awareness.

True healing is not about waiting for time to heal. It's about creating the environment where healing can take place. When you have a hobby or job that is part of your internal being and natural, God-given abilities, it's evident in your peace. We need health and wellness to build up our emotional strength so we can be open to inspiration—and therefore tap into our gifts.

advice to my younger self

In January of 2018, a friend reached out to me about her newly diagnosed celiac. She messaged me the news, and we scheduled a meet-up for the next day. I had 24 hours to think about what I was going to say, so I wrote her a letter. It got me thinking about how truly amazed I am with how my life has turned out even though I never thought that I would eventually be diagnosed with a food-based autoimmune disorder like celiac disease.

I wrote the letter as if I could go back in time to give advice to my younger self. This is what I shared with her:

Dear Adrienne,

I'm happy that I had 24 hours to think this through before we talked today. It helped me put together things I wish someone would've told me 15 years ago when I was first diagnosed with celiac disease. I'm grateful and humbled to be able to help you navigate your new diagnosis.

Here's the good part: You know now! That pesky piano you were carrying on your back while you were simultaneously doing everything else is now gone. And, there are no medications for you to take. It's only up from here.

The first lesson I can share with anyone in our shoes is this: You have to look out for yourself. The truth is that no one else has the fortitude and desire to help you navigate this gluten-free road as much as YOU do. It's not their fault. They have their own plates that need spinning. Often times we think, "Hey, what about ME? Throw me a lifeline. I'm unwell over here!" But, keeping their own shit together is their top priority, too. Life gets messy sometimes. We understand. Everyone is fighting their own battle, even though we may know nothing about it.

Coping with your new diagnosis is an mixture of emotions, maintenance and survival. My top three nuggets of wisdom for you are:

1. Stand tall
2. Self-care
3. Love yourself and will yourself well

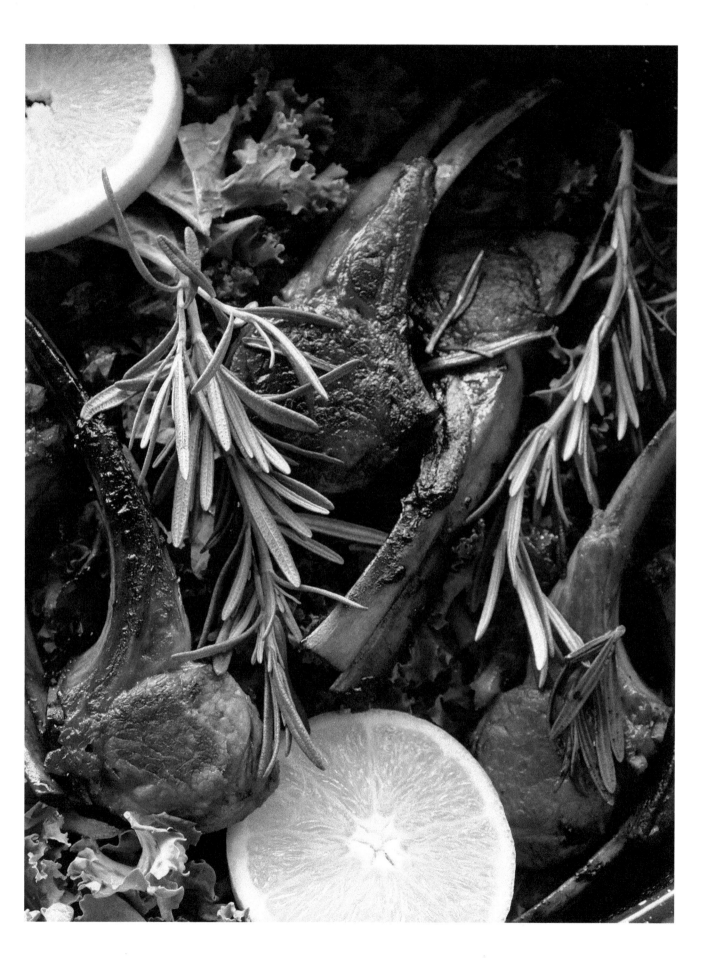

The problem with celiac disease is that it's tricky. It gets mislabeled. It's hard to pin down. One day it's one thing, and the next day, it's another. It's also difficult to diagnose because it affects people differently. There are more than 200 known celiac disease symptoms. Symptoms also vary depending on your age and the degree of damage to the small intestine.[46]

Doctors are human beings with many sick patients and limited time. I've learned that unless you're in immediate critical condition, your personal quality of life may not be their first focus. As it should be, saving lives is their first order of business—and, what a job that is. Working as a nurse has given me deep reverence for that. Once you can understand and appreciate that, you'll also be able to see why your achy joints at 30-years-old can't be on their top list of concerns and how your wellness and recovery has to *absolutely* be on the tippy-top of yours.

Now, on to the navigation of your current health situation:

- **First of all, drink a lot of water!**
  Hydration will help you on so many levels and is especially important for those recovering from malabsorption issues related to celiac disease and gluten intolerance. When your body is trying to heal itself, water is one of the best things to aid in the process.

- **Next, eat only single-ingredient, nutrient-dense foods.**
  It may be a tougher search to find things that sustain you if you're a vegetarian, but you have to persevere in order to feel fabulous. And, you will feel fabulous! This means fresh veggies, fruits, eggs, nuts and lean protein—all of which are delicious and healthful.

- **Ditch the dairy.**
  Don't wait like I did. There is all sorts of recent scientific research that ties lactose intolerance and celiac disease together.[47] Once I got rid of dairy and upped my water intake, I finally knew what true wellness could feel like.

- **Avoid all the overly processed, gluten-free replacements.**
  That stuff is full of sugar and hardcore-damaging ingredients that will take you down. I know you and can imagine that you give everything 100 percent of your effort. Trying to find the perfect cookie or muffin is not the best use of your precious time and energy.

  Gluten-free replacement foods wrecked me. I naively believed that these companies making alternatives to muffins and breads had some interest in my health and nutrition, but have now come to believe it's more of a monetary interest. Yes, there are healthy alternatives to gluten out there, but the simplest and most successful way to direct your energy is to eat the purest, freshest and most naturally colorful things you can find.

- **Get strong.**
  This is probably one of the most important things you can do, as your physical health and mental health are fundamentally linked.[48] Walk, lift light weights, dance, swim, sleep and build your strength doing things that you enjoy and make you feel good.

- **Focus on your recovery and gratitude.**
  Gratitude is imperative now that you know what you need to do. Don't weigh yourself down with the why's or the woulda-shoulda-coulda's. Your focus should instead be on being the best, most healthy version of yourself—in this moment, right NOW.

I'm so happy for you because you have a new year and a fresh start to this new life! I promise you that there is no material thing or gift that is bigger than your health. I love you and am here if you need me.

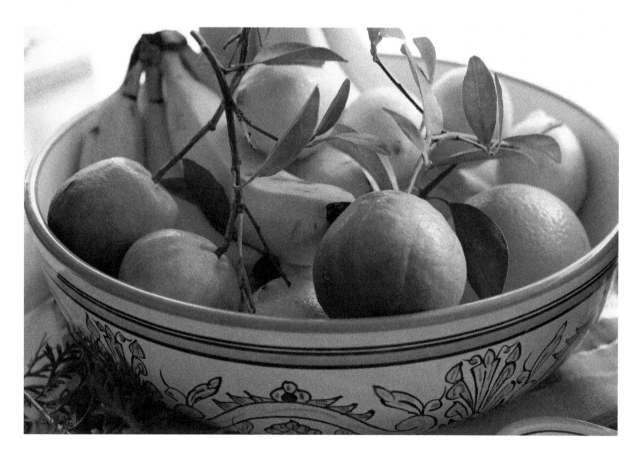

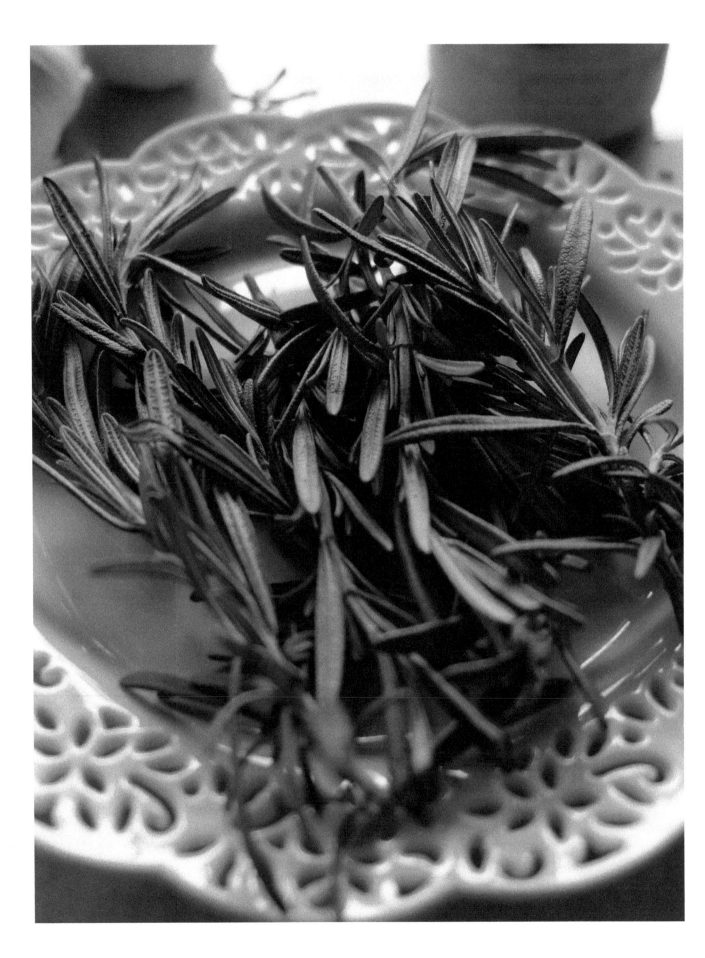

walk with the dreamers

I have a very clear memory surrounding my dream of hiking to the top of a mountain without stopping. Though I was young, thin and energetic, I could not hit my goal. I always visualized that I would make it. I made a clear workout plan to "stay ready so I ain't gotta get ready," however no preparation could get me there—because I had the silent version of celiac disease.

Silent celiac disease, or asymptomatic celiac disease, is celiac without obvious digestive symptoms. I was eating a healthy diet, but because I was also eating gluten, I wasn't able to absorb the goodness from my food, and was malnourished. I was anemic and always short of breath, yet cardiac work ups showed me in premium shape.

A year after my first son was born, I felt unreasonably exhausted and achy, and was haunted by migraines. I was dropping weight and my hair was thinning. Doctors told me that my brittle hair and fatigue were due to being a stressed-out mom; that my anemia was because I'm Italian.

Like many others with undiagnosed celiac, I lived for years with fatigue and unexplained symptoms, continually rationalizing them and telling myself to push on. It took 15 years of doctor visits and dangerously low iron levels before I was finally diagnosed.

How can someone eat gluten every day for decades without issue and then suddenly develop severe celiac disease symptoms? According to Dr. Amy Burkhart, celiac disease is hereditary, but there's something else needed to trigger the onset: an environmental factor. There is very little data available on the trigger(s) for celiac disease, but researchers have identified some possibilities including pregnancy, emotional or physical stress, menopause, antibiotic use, viruses and gastrointestinal infections.[46]

So basically: genes + gluten + trigger = celiac disease

Because celiac symptoms can be vague and mimic many other conditions, a diagnosis can be incorrect or missed altogether. In addition, blood test results for celiac disease may be normal even when you have the disease.

I was relieved and grateful for my diagnosis, but soon learned that healthful living with celiac is not only about diet. The gluten-free diet can be incredibly tricky to navigate at first since there's very little education available for learning about it, not to mention all the nutrient-deficient replacement foods out there.

Celiac disease is a hard thing to teach about or explain. If we all become more aware that food can be the reason we feel unwell, and if we're better educated about food-related illnesses, then many lives would be improved—whether one has celiac or not. If you know someone who feels tired, looks pale and either can't keep weight on or is gaining weight and can't lose it, they may have a food sensitivity. Encourage them to get tested. You might be the one who makes a difference in their existence.

If you think you may have celiac, have recently been diagnosed or have been struggling to find a new way of living around your diagnosis, please know that there are many resources and support out there for you to change your life in a way that brings power and strength into a healthy, feel-good and positive reality.

You can take further action to improve the health and well-being of the gluten-free communities through a variety of initiatives:

1. Make a donation to **Beyond Celiac** and/or the **Celiac Disease Foundation**. These organizations are forging pathways to improve quality of life for all people affected by gluten-related disorders and to find a cure for celiac disease. Your workplace may even have a matching gift program to double the impact of your gift.
2. Join the Celiac Disease Foundation's **Team Gluten Free** community fundraising program for a fun way to raise money and awareness!
3. Add your data to **iCureCeliac**, a patient-powered research network, which allows patients to contribute their own medical information and their experiences living with celiac disease and gluten sensitivity to help researchers improve treatments and find a cure.
4. Become a Celiac Disease Foundation **Patient Advocate** to help design and evaluate celiac disease research.
5. Join a celiac disease **Support Group**.[47]
6. Get tested! If a family member is diagnosed with celiac disease there's a 1-in-20 chance that a first-degree relative like a parent, child or sibling will also get celiac disease, and a 1-in-39 chance for second-degree relatives such as aunts, uncles and grandparents.[48]

Trust your gut and keep going until you get answers. I changed my life, and you can too. As hard as it may be, take good care of yourself and keep dreaming. Having hope is a necessity and can help you adjust, make a roadmap and clearly see the path that stretches out before you. The dreamers I know do big stuff. Great, big stuff. I think they go hand in hand.

The caretakers
The promise keepers
The dream weavers
The sincere believers

I admire these positively positive people. I dream of them surrounding me and being as dreamy as they are every single day. I'm following in your footsteps, folks!

A good attitude is important, but action paired with a positive mindset is essential. I learn from my friends how to stay positive, dream large and keep my chin up. You've got a bad shoulder, but still put on a happy grin. Now we're talking. You're juggling multiple roles and responsibilities, but people are expecting you, so you show up. That's some big dedication to this life's mission. You have a life-threatening illness, and you're still next-level stoic. Now you've blown my mind.

After trying several possibilities and learning from those outcomes, I finally figured out the balance of diet and exercise that keeps me energized, happy, and thankfully, healthy. My dreams of hiking the long trail were fulfilled. Being in high altitudes, taking in deep breaths of fresh mountain air and feeling well is magical.

I went for it. And though it may be a small milestone to some, it meant a lot to me. You see, dreams can be big or small. Endless kindness even in the midst of chaos. Smiles even in the face of adversity. I'm cheering for you, as I imagine you are for me.

You are amazing and beautiful, and the world needs you to be healthy. Each and every gorgeous day, take very good care of yourself. Learn from me. I am your gluten-free, lab-tested being! I am so grateful to be able to support your health. The more people out there who can find this path as soon as they've been diagnosed with celiac, the better they will be.

Never give up on you. It's not selfish; it's a *necessity*. Your tribe needs YOU.

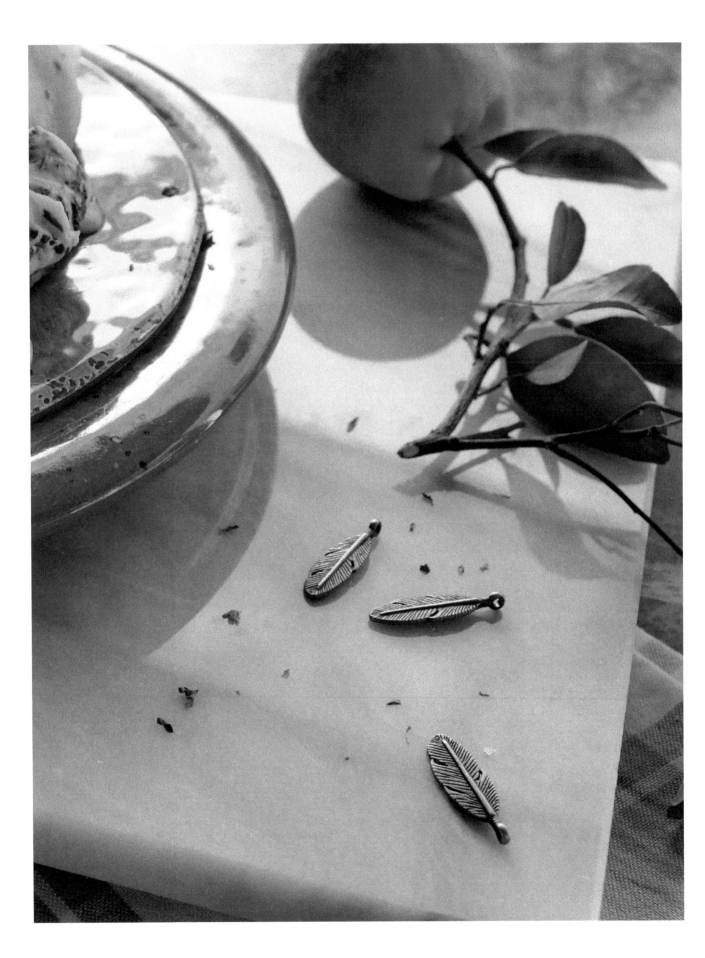

Inspiration: Thrust

"Thrust is the force that's generated by an aircraft's propulsion system to counteract drag and move the aircraft through the air. When the forces of thrust and drag are equal, the aircraft is balanced and flies at constant airspeed. When thrust is greater than drag, the aircraft is able to accelerate and climb. Powered by the aircraft's engine, the propeller creates a difference in air pressure between the front and back of the propeller blades and pulls the aircraft forward."

Air in Motion: Aerodynamics and the Four Forces of Flight from Hartzell Propeller, Inc.

why inspiration matters

In September of 2016, I wrote a blog post about inspiration and why inspiration matters. It began with happy memories of the pop-culture years of the late '60s and how they kept showing up throughout my days—either as a wistful thought or nostalgic feeling. This seemed like too much of a coincidence. I wanted to investigate further. As I did, more synchronicities occurred, and I found myself suddenly following an exciting line of action and reaction. My soul was sending me on a journey.

Inspiration is so incredibly important and is the springboard for creativity. I didn't realize the true impact of this until I became well. These past few years have been transformative for me. Primarily because I discovered that there's a process one must go through to open oneself up to inspiration and take meaningful action around it. The simplest way I learned to do this was by taking care of myself.

There is a time in my life that I refer to as "building my cathedral". This refers to the time when I was navigating my pre-celiac diagnosis while working as a nurse and raising my family. Raising my boys was everything to me. I took the job seriously and was incredibly focused.

Something I learned a couple of years ago from Danielle LaPorte's *Desire Map* is how to use my core desired feelings as a guidance system for goal setting. We all have an emotional guidance system. For example, how do you want to feel when you hike a mountain? When I was first diagnosed with celiac, I could barely get to the top of the two flights of stairs to my husband's office. I would get to the top, put my hand on the doorknob and catch my breath.

The turning point was in 2015 when I walked 4.6 miles up to Booth Falls in Vail, Colorado. From having a tough time climbing two flights of stairs to being able to scale 1000 feet was a monumental improvement! I skipped down the mountain with a great sense of accomplishment and satisfaction—a direct result of changing my diet and lifestyle.

I'm an adventurous girl at heart, and my emotional guidance system was tugging at my conscience and reminding me of this. My climb up to Booth Falls is symbolic of my ascent up the emotional mountain of feeling weak and discouraged, to hopeful and optimistic. These new, positive expectations and beliefs led me to additional interests in hiking, swimming,

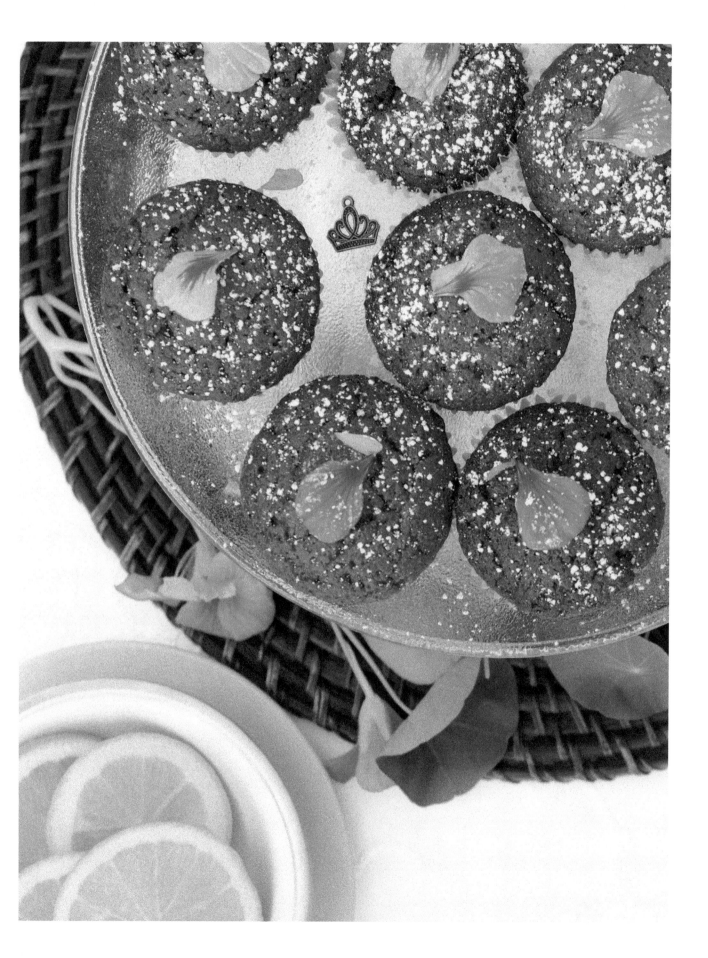

nature and poetry, all of which have become passions of mine.

At some point in our life, many of us stop trusting or following our own guidance—and for various reasons. The truth is that you're the only one who truly knows who you are and what you need—whether it's to heal your body, follow your purpose or whatever your heart desires. Listen to your emotions. Learning to trust and follow your own guidance will support you 100 percent in making positive changes in all areas of your life and helping you to heal.

Inspiration can be activated, captured and used to motivate, and has a major effect on important life outcomes. Every day, I continue to wake up with my shoulders back and a "go get 'em" attitude; a new, improved state of mind and self-care. It's not just work, work, work anymore, but instead, is an awesome balance of helping others while doing what makes me feel good. So, the more I eat well, exercise and write poetry, the more I feel inspired. The more open I am to inspiration, the more open I am to new possibilities.

If you have a big dream that your heart truly desires, don't let anything stop you. Sure, it's risky. But if you can make a difference and possibly change people's lives, then you have to march forward and DO IT. I've learned this by living it; by watching people before me, by risking criticism, by wearing my heart on my sleeve and by making sacrifices and going full-out-on-a-limb. I know the concept of risk is relative and that the tolerance for it is in the eye of the beholder, but I believe that for the value I receive, it's worth it.

My illustrated poetry book *Wild White Indigo* is one of those risks, but it's also why inspiration matters. I didn't set out with the intention of publishing a third book. I just wrote. I tweeted micropoetry. I texted rhyming messages to friends and family. I thought of poems at the gas pump, when opening a bottle of wine and on hikes while walking among native wildflowers. I showed up every day and put in the effort, driven by the desire to do what I love.

White Wild Indigo is an accumulation of all these bits and bursts of inspiration, poetry and synchronicity, brought to life by the beautiful and talented Annie Moor. It was upon meeting Annie that I decided on a third book, inspired by her and her art.

This book serves as an important reminder to live in the present moment, appreciating all that I have and all the beauty that surrounds me. Poetry has opened doors to meaningful relationships and experiences. It has made me more aware of my own intuitive thoughts,

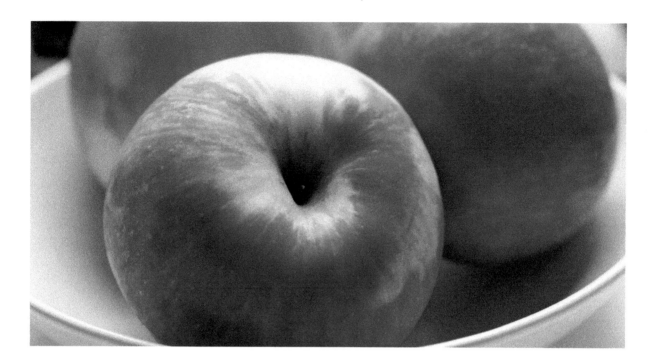

which may suggest a course of action to move my life forward with passion and determination.

If something changes your life and you do something differently because of it, then that experience changes your motivations. Motivations are emotions. The more something has value, meaning, purpose or importance, the more it motivates you. My celiac diagnosis certainly changed my life. It taught me how to identify and treat the cause of what was making me feel bad. It motivated me to create a website as a platform for healthy living through artful experiences and a voice for those whose bodies and spirits needed healing.

Human beings need to have something that they are committed to and passionate about; something that can be directed toward helping others or the world. I believe that trusting that your life has purpose will give you resiliency. When something stressful comes along, you'll able to handle it better because you have things in your life that give your life meaning and purpose.

I've learned that taking action on inspiration and giving your whole self to your purpose is one of the greatest joys in life—from both the successes and failures. So, take the risk. It's too risky NOT to.

your mass is critical

I had an important errand to run. It was pretty far away, but it had to be done. I hopped in Jade, my beautiful Ford truck. I was thinking, "Whew… this will be a trek," but I was determined to make the best of it. I put on Otis Redding's *The Happy Song*, and both the song and Jade got me through.

I adopted Jade out of my love for the tough, the rugged and the exquisite. I wanted a truck to protect me—one that I could keep forever. An ol' pal I could listen to music with and who can take me wherever I need to go. She has no choice but to love the tiny bits of inspiration I bring to her with unconditional love. Yes, I know, I'm talking about my truck. I've never been so enamored by a thing before, that I wrote a poem about her:

I don't like material things
But your presence gives me a serious zing
Makes my heart go ring-a-ling
My love is everlasting—I'll keep you 'til you're old and gray
But I want you while you're young today

I arrived at my destination, and the music and mindset did the trick. All emotion comes from our thoughts, so if we change our thoughts, our thoughts will then change our emotions—a chain reaction. My newfound wave of enthusiasm was carried over when I went inside and ran into a long-time acquaintance. I was there to drop something off, but who knew that he would impart the best wisdom of the day to me.

We talked about a mutual friend whom we both love who had moved away. I told him about my poetry books. He told me about his personal poetry and how he had previously stopped writing, but recently picked it up again. I told him that he had to keep at it—that life is too short to leave the call of our purpose unanswered. He said I wasn't the first person to tell him this and shared a story with me that had reignited his fire of inspiration.

He then took a carpenter's tape measure out of his pocket and created a beautiful analogy of how a tape measure can represent a life span. He asked me what I thought was the average life span of a person in the U.S., and I answered, "Eighty." He pulled the tape measure out to 80" to represent an average life expectancy of 80 years old. Then, he put his finger on the number of his age to show how many years have passed and how many years there are left to go until he reaches the age of 80.

To see it visually in this way gave me some perspective. I saw that he was trying to illustrate my point, showing me how each one of us has to take advantage of each and every day we have. We need to strive to be conscious of our purpose and pursue it. Why should we wait? Why stop doing anything we love dearly and deeply?

A life inspired by purpose is a life defined by meaning. When you have something important and meaningful to work toward, you will be more engaged and fulfilled by life's pursuits. What once appeared to be risky now becomes a path you feel compelled to follow because you are following your bliss, which is the truth within you.

You can design your environment to increase your life's satisfaction regardless of your age, who or where you are, and what you do for a living. Make your surroundings conducive to the warmth and purity needed to write, paint or play your instrument. Let your passion and purpose take shape. Spend time doing things that speak to your heart. Understand what gives you energy, so you can create a life that fills you up. It's all about knowing what's critical to your mass.

For a physicist, a critical mass is the smallest amount of fissile material needed for a sustained nuclear chain reaction. The critical mass of this material depends upon its properties, its density, its shape, its enrichment, its purity, its temperature and its surroundings. Similarly, we have our own ability to achieve a self-sustaining reaction under certain conditions.

It's easy to embrace inspiration when we're children. Our daily work is to stay creative, engaged, laughing, learning and curious.

What conditions do you need in order to explode into being and further your growth? Take care of your body. Get plenty of sleep. Disconnect from your smart phone or social media. Set up your bedroom so it's a relaxing environment to sleep in. Develop a new hobby. Sing. Dance. Draw. Paint. Write. Exercise. Eat better. Plant a garden. Get outdoors. Write poetry. Design the life that will give you good health, a sense of purpose, satisfaction and well-being.

Whatever you must do to make your spirit soar, do it. Your mass is critical. Watch the chain reaction and feel the fullness it brings you. Your soul will thank you.

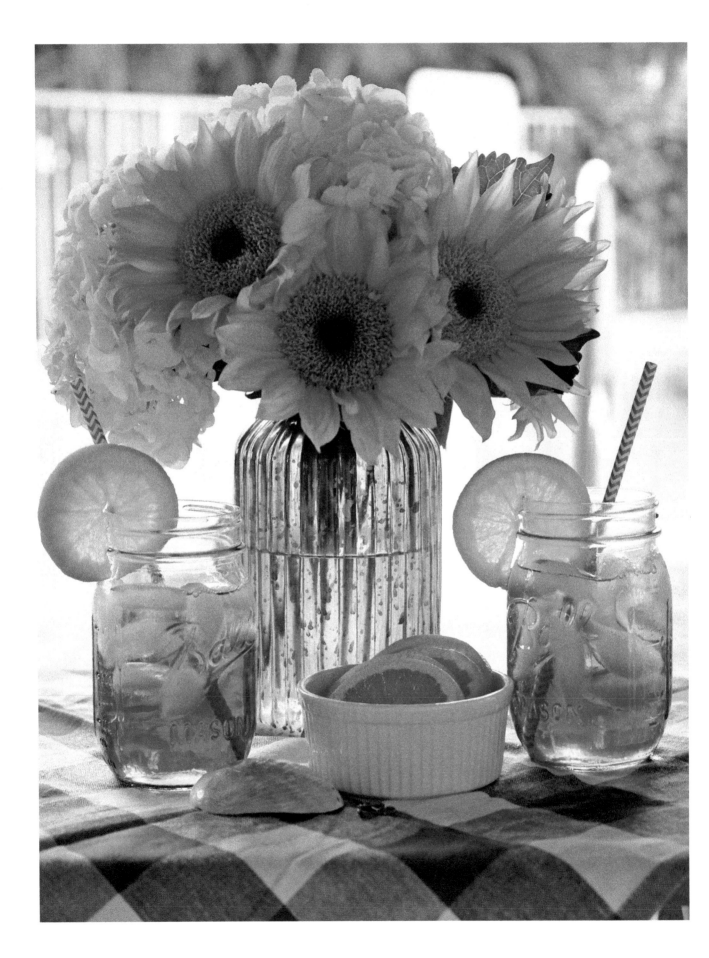

catalyst for happiness

There are some things that stick with you and will always leave a smile on your face when you reminisce about your travels. For me, it's the people moments. Dinner conversations around the table on topics like paying attention to the universe and its messages, raising kids and—one of my personal favorites, TED Talks—really get me jazzed.

Someone recommended that I watch one on *The Boiling River of the Amazon* by geoscientist Andres Ruzo. Talk about loving life, curiosity and contagious happiness. Ruzo has this tenfold. The subject matter—the existence of the boiling river, its history and the science behind it—is also fascinating. Because he loves his work, Ruzo is exhilarating to watch. He found his life's joy in his work through studying this natural phenomenon and how it came to be.

What's the significance? It's sacred.

I think about the boiling river and compare it to life. And though some might exploit this land, it's important to keep this from happening or to keep it from becoming trivial. It's important to protect its purity and natural state. I wish for each and every person to have the same honor and integrity for themselves that Ruzo feels for the Amazon.

I'm all about using good judgment. It's something my mom and dad instilled in me throughout my childhood. Critical thinking, proper assessment and good judgment skills are all lessons I also learned in nursing school. Good judgment isn't about being smart. It's about reflection, learning from past mistakes and applying feedback to the next opportunity. It's about remaining open, and understanding that unexpected outcomes are a real and likely occurrence.

To use good judgment is to be reasonably prudent. A reasonably prudent person is defined as "someone who uses good judgment or common sense in handling practical matters. The actions of a person exercising common sense in a similar situation are the guide in determining whether an individual's actions were reasonable." This definition has stuck with me throughout my life.

I believe being reasonably prudent leads to peace and happiness. You simplify and therefore make life as smooth as you can. I don't know one single person who likes stress. I personally, as a mother, daughter, friend, partner and responsible adult, like to stick to the wild flowers—not the wild goose chase. The long hike, not the ice pick climb. The Rocky Mountains instead of Everest. It's my personal preference and what brings me joy.

Once we reasonably tend to our responsibilities, we free ourselves up for the goodies of life! During a trip to Washington D.C. with all obligations out of the way, I found myself on the water with the sails up and engine off. I then turned off my phone. Now I'm watching a river and quietly contemplating the meaning of a TED Talk. Which brings me to psychology professor Dan Gilbert's talk on *The Surprising Science of Happiness* and the study that he did.

Gilbert brings to the forefront of my mind what happens when a person can take life too far and be reckless or unbound—to go on the hike without water or necessary gear, for example—and what that does to someone's mind and sense of happiness. He explains it so well.

Why do people do the things they do? How is it that some people live and breathe happiness, while others seem to constantly be in an elusive pursuit of it? According to Gilbert, there are two kinds of happiness: One is **natural happiness** which we experience when we get what we want, and the other is **synthetic happiness** which we manufacture when we don't get what we want. Natural happiness lets us relish in the good stuff while synthetic happiness lets us adapt and appreciate what we do have when the outcome is less than ideal.

Yes, some things are better than others. We should have a freedom of choice that leads us into one future over another. But as Gilbert explains, when those preferences drive us too hard and too fast—when we have overrated the differences between these futures—we are at risk. When our ambition is bounded, it leads us to work joyfully. When our ambition is unbounded, it leads us to sacrifice things of real value.[49]

Most people want to be unencumbered by the heavy weights this life can sometimes bring. Gilbert teaches us that synthetic happiness is just as real and enduring as natural happiness. He also teaches us that our longings and worries are overblown because we have the capacity to create a catalyst for happiness within ourselves, rather than depend on experiences to make us happy. The best part? He tells us the very condition under which synthetic happiness grows.

Synthetic happiness is every bit as real and enduring as the kind of happiness you experience when you get exactly what you were aiming for. When we have choices, we worry about lost opportunity. When we don't have choices, we come to like what we've got, more than what we originally predicted.

Nobody wants to disrupt the future tranquility of their mind. We want to be resilient enough to be able to fully handle the true, gritty part of our experiences; something that should be taught from a very young age and serve as a reminder throughout our lives. Peacefulness, hence happiness, is not trivial. It's sacred.

Here's a point to ponder: An illness that once made me afraid to eat, has led me to discover a love for food—and life.

I can attest that pure wellness and a healthy diet lead to inner strength and a sense of peace, which gives one the ability to spend time outdoors and build an exercise routine. This leads to feeling good, and—you guessed it—happy. Then inspiration follows, and the ability to follow through with your creative projects falls right in line. It's a domino effect.

A joyful life is not always about getting what you want but learning to enjoy what you get. If you know that you can be happy both by getting what you want as well as when you don't, it can take the pressure off of feeling like you have something to prove to the world. Enjoying something without feeling deprived or defeated has to go hand in hand with the ability to take charge of your life and go after the things that are important to you.

"Happiness always looks small while you hold it in your hands, but let it go, and you learn at once how big and precious it is."
– Maxim Gorky, writer, author and political activist

I feel that both of these two very different TED Talks come from the same place. Good judgment, which ties in with overall wellness. Kindness and gratitude, which opens our hearts and minds to bring us joy through tough times. Integrity and effort, which creates happiness.

Each one of us has within us the capacity to manufacture the very thing we're constantly chasing when we choose an experience. We can't control the world, but we can do our darndest to share goodness every day—to know what we value, to love deeply and to express our appreciation. These are the things that make people happy. Real life. Go out and touch it.

sacred spaces

My favorite time of day is first light—the time in early morning hours when light first appears and before the sun rises. When you're all alone in the morning, you're able to consciously embrace the calm and the quiet all around you. This silence allows you to focus on self-reflection and opens you up for inspiration. I feel like each day's first light is precious. I wake early just to savor this sacred moment.

One weekend, I caught it under a canopy-covered road in north central Florida on my way to a secret birding spot that a naturalist had shared with me in confidence. It's light was streaming through a tunnel of trees. We went to see swallow-tailed kites by the hundreds right as they take their first drink of the morning. We arrived at our location in time to see the sunrise, and it was spectacular. It's one of my new favorite places and spaces, and a precious day for my heart to hold on to forever. I'm incredibly grateful for these sacred spaces that inspire awe and wonder in my life because I've spent so many years running and hustling through my days.

I haven't always been looking at birds and enjoying first light. There have been times when I was incredibly focused on the health and safety of my children. Here's an example to illustrate the point: Birds are singing overhead trying to capture your attention and greet you with a big "Hello!" You barely see or hear them as you diligently buckle your child's car seat into the car. Your attention to detail is a necessity and not something you take lightly. You want to look up, but your focus is on the most important thing in that moment; those tiny hands and bright eyes looking up at you as you get ready for the big day ahead. You're asking yourself, "Did the backpacks and lunches make it to the car? Is the coffeepot off? Is everyone alive and healthy? Ok, mission accomplished."

Raising my boys was the most courageous and rewarding job I've ever had, but let's be honest. Parenting is difficult. The boys were not the challenge, though. It was navigating the world as a family—and through an illness—that was the true test of strength and character.

I was working in survival mode and focusing all my energy on the next task ahead of me (never mind the next week or even the next year). When you're in the "messy middle," looking out the window (or heck, even the mirror) is not on the priority list. Before you know it, it's nighttime and you've missed the new roses popping up or the cardinal couple at the bird feeder.

Survival mode can happen as a result of an illness or trauma, but it can also happen during a move, job changes, pregnancy and birth, or while parenting. What I've learned about survival mode is that it keeps you outside of your life. This is not healthy or sustainable for many reasons. Most importantly, with the lack of connection to yourself comes a lack of self-care; which means we don't eat well, we don't exercise and we don't sleep regularly or enough.

Self-care is your sacred space. Sacred spaces are environments that protect, nourish and provide inspiration. They give us a place to slow down for creative thought and reflection. They give us the space to reconnect with ourselves and just be. So many of us give to our families unceasingly, and to the neglect of our own health and well-being. Sacred spaces can help us pause, unplug and reflect on the work that really matters. Making space in your life for taking care of yourself is key. It takes practice, but once it becomes a priority, it comes naturally and spontaneously. We then become appreciative for our responsibilities and the joyful things life has given us.

There will be times in your life when just getting through the day is your main goal. These are the days when you need self-care the most. If you only had a few minutes to spend in your sacred space every day, what would that look like? Maybe it's a peaceful and uncluttered area in your home. Maybe it's 10 minutes of solitude in the quiet of the morning before the rest of the house wakes up. It could be closing your eyes and listening to the rain falling or thinking of a memory that holds a cherished place in your heart.

Find encouraging, inspiring, empowering messages throughout your day. Turn them up! All the things you do become what you are. Find your own sacred space and make it yours to keep. It's precious to your soul for you to take the time to appreciate your daily efforts, determination, and dedication. Know what you need to make it work and always give it your best.

Respect and loyalty to a project is where the peace of mind comes in. Instead of frantic action, focus on the sacred and the exact thing you are doing in the present moment. Let go of the things that don't matter and hold on to the essential. You are enough. Tomorrow, you will be enough too.

disconnect to reconnect

I took a weeklong trip through the country of Cuba at the beginning of 2018. Living off the grid has taken on an entirely new meaning to me. When I left home, it didn't occur to me that I wouldn't have access to email, text messaging or WiFi for that matter. Data didn't work on my phone the entire time I was there and internet access wasn't easy to find, or convenient. I had to log on at a telecommunications center (Empresa de Telecomunicaciones de Cuba S.A.) or at a hotel with WiFi accessibility and buy a card to access it.

I love being in constant communication with my boys as well as staying on top of current events. But these past three years, I've found myself on my phone and computer more and more while writing and launching my website, my poetry and this book.

Now that my sons are grown men and so near to each other, I feel they have each other to call if either of them needs help in any way. Because of this, I worried less about my off-line status while traveling and decided after my first day there to put the phone down and disconnect. I'd found myself desiring a digital detox of sorts for a while now but hadn't pulled the plug until the situation presented itself. This meant not using the phone's camera either.

Being without WiFi for a week, I learned how simply we can live. Either by choice, or necessity. The detox was a blessing in disguise. No longer controlled by the urgency of the moment, I had time on my hands to observe and reflect while surrounded by beautiful people and scenery. I observed those around me who seemed as if they did not have much to do, but realized that this leisure time gave way for creativity and deliberateness of thought, and a little more space for daydreaming.

When you tuck your phone and laptop out of sight for a week, you become overwhelmed—by a feeling of peace. You notice the birds singing and the rain on the roof. Your focus is spot-on as you engage more meaningfully in your surroundings with all your heart.

One afternoon, we stumbled upon a guitarist on a restaurant patio whistling as he strummed. I most likely would've pulled out my phone and recorded this priceless moment, only to later

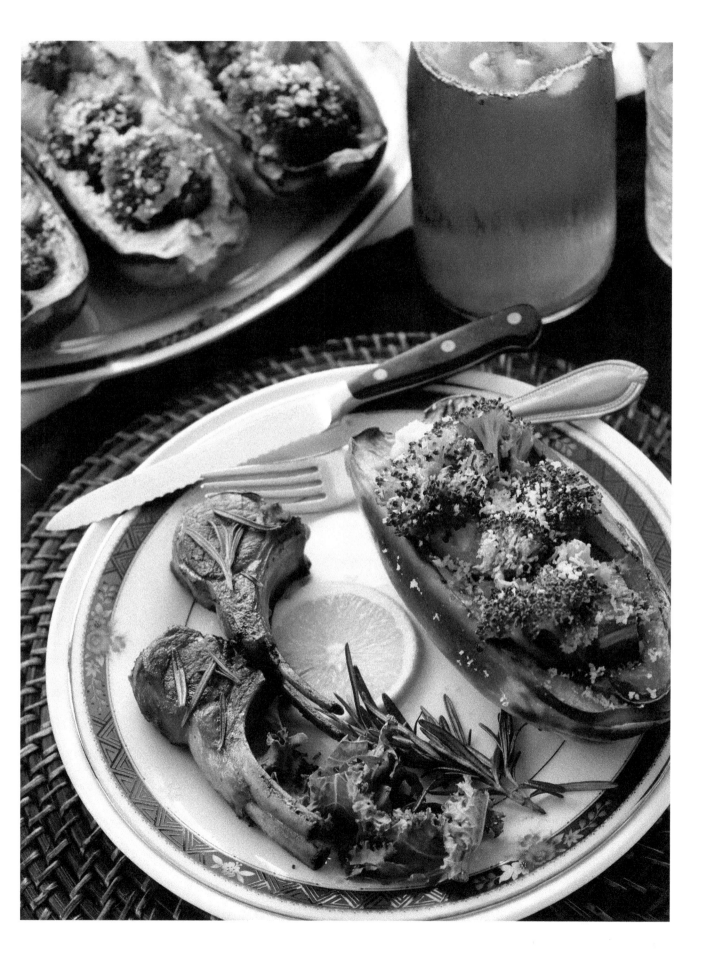

discover that the picture was shaky and the sound quality so bad that it wasn't worth reliving, or even keeping. Instead, I watched and listened with all my senses—no screen in between. I was living in the moment and feeding off of his energy and that of the restaurant instead of trying to capture it. There was some beautiful bougainvillea cascading behind him with the sun streaming down. It was the sweetest sound on earth.

Another unintentional disconnect-to-reconnect was when I learned that I could not use credit cards in Cuba, only cash. I was reminded of how simple and efficient it is to pay for something as you use or need it. You become more aware of what you're spending, as it frees you up to be more in the moment. I believe we can value and appreciate it more this way, too.

Upon my return home to Florida, I bought a copy of Outdoor Life's *Live Off The Grid*. And though I'm very happy and grateful to be back in my home country, my perspective has shifted and curiosity piqued. During my time away, I detoxed on technology and "stuff" in a major way. I learned a lot from the freedom from my societal norms and the idea of loosening my ties to modern consumer culture.

There seems to be a current homesteading trend and desire to live off-grid as more people shift to a simpler and more mindful way of living. However, it's a major lifestyle change to truly live off-grid in the traditional homesteading fashion. The idea of living in a lil' farmhouse in the woods with an organic garden and chicken coop out back sounds romantic and dreamy at times, but instead I'd like to bring the essence of what I learned in Cuba back to my everyday life in a way that's practical and realistic. I found a wonderful explanation by author Abigail R. Gehring of what this could mean:

"Homesteading is about creating a lifestyle that is, first of all, genuine. It's about learning to recognize your needs—including energy, food, financial, and health needs—and finding out how they can be met creatively and responsibly." – from *Pacific Standard* magazine

Many people opting to go off the grid aim for a healthy and wholesome lifestyle. This includes sticking to a natural diet and avoiding processed foods. Some people do it to be self-reliant or more in touch with nature. I've found that when I make a conscious effort to eat whole, nutrient-dense foods and regularly connect with nature in some way, that I am much more energized, productive, creative and inspired in my work and life.

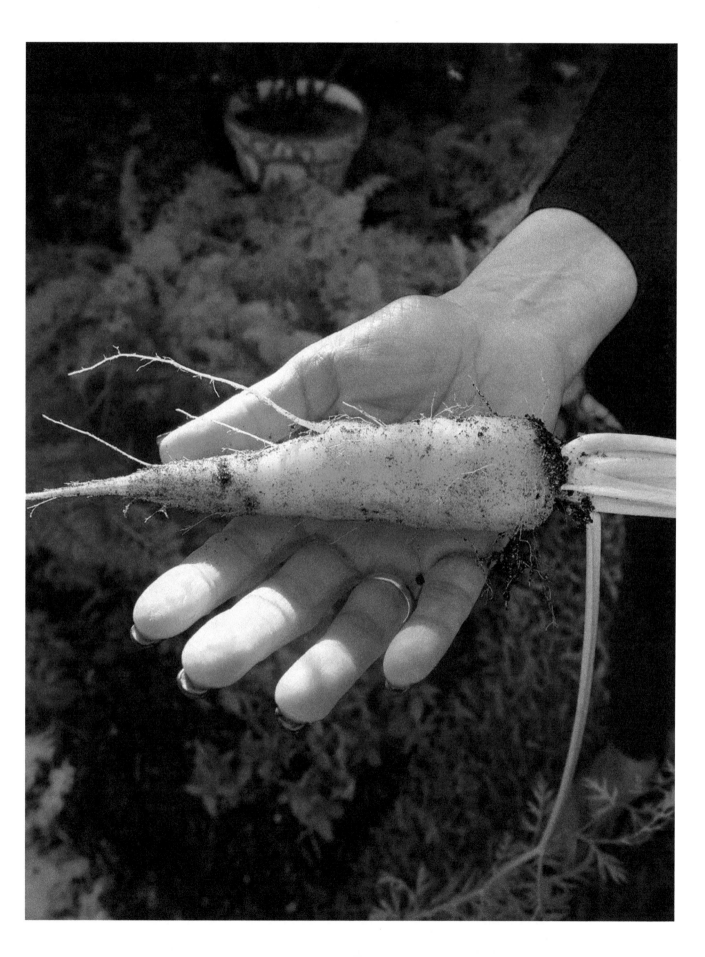

Being outside is my love. It's the trustworthy partner of my dreams; reliable, intriguing, interesting and always there to love me up unconditionally. Whether it's stargazing, catching a moonrise, watching meteor showers or the Hubble Space Telescope in the sky above, all are better than anything I could watch on T.V. Nature will quiet your mind, open your heart and invite ease into your body. It gives me that peaceful, easy feeling, fills me with endless gratitude and keeps me well. It's one of my reasons to wake up each day.

According to Dr. John Swartzberg at U.C. Berkeley: "The proposed benefits of walking in nature include giving the brain a respite from the multitasking of everyday life. If you enjoy hiking, you know that you become more aware of your surroundings—the sounds, smells, colors. Time slows down. Somehow this refreshes the brain and makes thinking clearer. All it takes is five to 20 minutes in nature to boost mood and energy levels somewhat, though longer forays produce greater benefits. Other studies indicate that there's a 'third-day effect'—a special stage of relaxation and mindfulness that occurs after a couple days of hiking."[49]

My love of walking and hiking is one thing, but at the same time, *everything* to me. It's one of the most accessible and easiest forms of exercise! It could be a city park, by the shore or on a backroad trail. Be curious and discover what kind of environmentalist you are. The health benefits of walking are endless and it beats any gym.

There are many things you can do to easily bring the essence of homesteading to your life in practical, everyday ways:

- Plant wildflowers in your yard or garden and gather them to put inside your home in a vase. Admire the beautiful colors.
- Start a veggie or herb garden. Plant a fruit tree. If you don't have a green thumb, start a windowsill garden and see what grows from there. A windowsill garden is a great way to bring color and texture to a room.
- Enjoy a cup of coffee or tea outside. Savor every sip and soak up the fresh air.
- Walk barefoot on the grass or along the beach. Focus on the sense of feeling grounded that can come along with this.
- Take short breaks from your work to go outside. Be still. Notice things about your environment that you've never seen before. Actively examine the trees, the clouds, the birds, the air and any other sights, smells and sounds.
- Move your body in the great outdoors for a while. Pick a park and go for a walk, run or

hike. Fresh air and sun exposure are just a couple of examples of how getting outside each day can improve your connection to nature and your overall health.

- Google your zipcode and search for new places and walks for you to explore. You can find the most fantastic bird trails, butterflies, flowers and wildlife—right in your own city, county or neighborhood. You'll be pleasantly surprised!
- Buy indoor plants or flowers to add color and greenery to your house or workspace.
- Open your windows, and even doors, to allow sunlight and fresh air to flow through your home for a more relaxing and natural atmosphere.
- Eat more whole, nutrient-dense foods. Eating foods that were naturally grown or raised works wonders for your health and well-being.
- Shop at your local farmer's market. Knowing your food is naturally produced allows you to savor each meal with confidence in your ingredients.
- Disconnect to reconnect. Switch off technology and enjoy the great outdoors for a while. Listen to the birds, the wind, the rain or the waves. Enjoy the stillness.
- Make an effort to spend time by the water. Go swimming, dip your toes in the ocean or float in a local river or lake for a while. Water is the fundamental basis of all life on Earth and is naturally soothing to our souls!
- Stargazing and watching the night sky is a humbling way to admire the universe and all of its possibilities. There's something incredibly magical about this.
- Find your sacred space where you can escape the cacophony. Get in touch with your feelings and listen to your heart.

My takeaway from this experience is to embrace inspiration from everything around you. When you're not looking down at a screen, you look up! And when you remember to look up, you stand taller, breathe deeper and take it all in. Everything. There isn't much required of us to have beautiful moments and maintain health, if we are so fortunate to have it.

Take regular breaks from technology to check-in with your emotional self and take care of your soul. Tune into the beauty of creation. Do what you can, when you can. Be mindful of how you use your resources. Practice in your own backyard. Whatever it takes to create a meaningful and healthy life.

Inspiration is EVERYWHERE. You have to be present to see it. If you're consumed by technology and the self-imposed responsibilities of being connected, you're going to miss all the beauty that surrounds you.

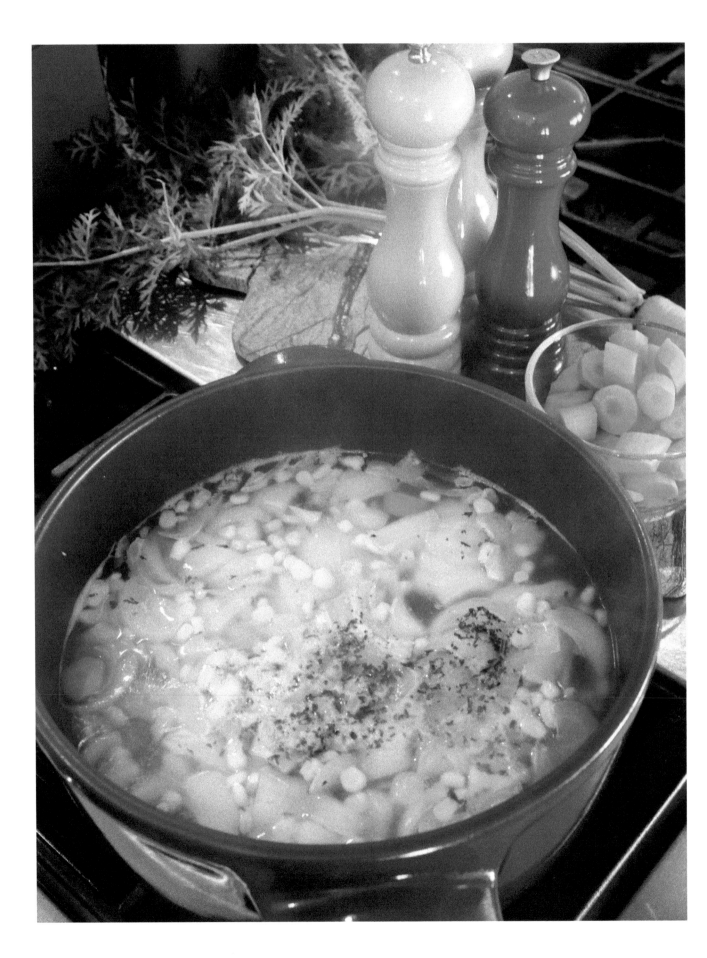

3

recipes

*Premium fuel to be healthy, radiant
and bounding with energy.*

My training is my own personal and lifelong
experience in an Italian-American kitchen
mixed with learning how to eat for celiac
disease through the gluten-free diet.

rosemary lamb chops with orange slices

These rosemary lamb chops with orange slices are super simple. There isn't really a true recipe for these, but below is a general rule of thumb to follow when making them. You can use Australian or Colorado single cut lamb chops. Both are delicious, but I prefer the chops from Colorado. The colors will be poppin' and your kitchen will smell like a dream.

Heat olive oil in a large skillet over medium heat. Add lamb chops to skillet and sprinkle with chopped rosemary.

Slice the Navel oranges and place them in the same pan as the lamb chops.

Cook to desired doneness turning until evenly cooked through, about 3 minutes per side for medium-rare.

Transfer to platter and garnish with fresh rosemary sprigs and kale, if desired. I like to squeeze a dash of key lime on them, too.

Pair them up with a side of oven roasted potatoes and Brussels sprouts for a special, easy dinner.

8 single cut lamb chops

2 tablespoons chopped fresh rosemary

3 tablespoons extra virgin olive oil

2 Naval oranges

2-3 kale leaves, chopped in large pieces

Fresh rosemary sprigs (optional)

Extra virgin olive oil

Salt and pepper to taste

Serves 4–6

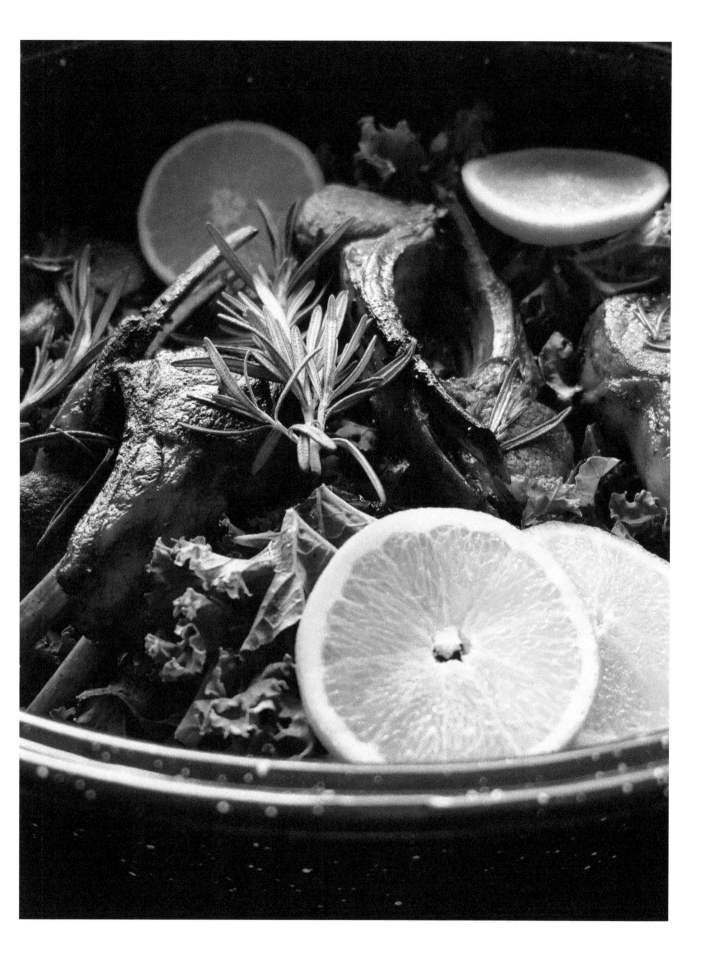

cuban pulled pork stuffed avocados

I have seven avocado trees that I grew from seeds, so my love for avocados is immense. I'll eat gluten-free anything with an avocado, so this recipe was super fun to make, though the plating was a bit of a challenge. My inspiration came from a favorite local Cuban restaurant, Havana, in West Palm Beach. I ordered their Lechón Asado, which is roasted pork, pulled and grilled, with fresh sautéed onions and a touch of Havana's signature mojo sauce. I made my own version at home with barbeque sauce, and oh my was it good.

Place pork roast in a slow cooker and rub with the olive oil, garlic, salt and pepper. Add sliced onion and chicken broth.

Set crock pot to high for 4 hours.

Remove the roast and onion from the slow cooker and place in 13×9 glass Pyrex dish allowing the meat to cool. Then begin pulling it apart with 2 forks or your fingers, discarding any fat along the way.

Toss the pulled pork and onions in the Pyrex with some of the pan drippings to keep it moist, then add the BBQ sauce of your choice.

Bake in the oven at 400º for 15 minutes to get the edges of the pork nice n' crispy.

Top each avocado half with pulled pork, then sprinkle with sweet peas and chopped cilantro.

You can substitute baked potatoes for the avocados and scoop out the centers to fill up with the pork, peas and cilantro for a heartier version of the recipe.

4 pounds pork shoulder/Boston butt pork roast

4 cups of chicken broth

3 cloves garlic, peeled and pressed

2 tablespoons extra virgin olive oil

Salt and pepper

1 sweet onion, sliced

Bone-Suckin' Sauce, or your favorite gluten-free BBQ sauce

4–6 ripe Florida or Haas avocados, seeded and cut in halves

2 cups sweet peas, steamed

¼ cup fresh cilantro, chopped (optional)

Serves 6–8

simple boil and bake barbeque ribs

There's nothing quite like Texas BBQ. I had some of the best food I've EVER eaten the last time I was in Texas, so one Memorial Day Weekend I planned a full-out BBQ rib dinner. I've made ribs more times than I can count, but the time before this they didn't turn out quite like I wished. I was in a hurry and any wise culinarian knows that you can't rush good barbeque! I finally got up the courage to make 'em again, and it was well worth the wait. Spot-on fall-off-the-bone pork BBQ ribs with Stubbs Hickory Bourbon barbeque sauce. They were a hit!

Boil ribs on medium heat for 2 hours, uncovered.

Preheat oven to 375º. Place ribs meat-side down in a glass Pyrex casserole dish.

Apply coating of salt and pepper to all sides of rib rack and add sauce to cover.

Bake for 30 minutes. Remove and cool for 10 minutes.

Cut rack into individual rib segments and serve with more barbeque sauce!

---

1 large slab (approx 3 lbs) pork baby back ribs

1 jar of Stubb's BBQ sauce (their hickory bourbon is the perfect amount of smoky and sweet)

Salt and pepper to taste

Serves 4–6

veggie prep
for the perfect stew
comfort food
for me and you
greets you
when your day is through!

– jet –

pork roast with root vegetables

This started out as an ambitious Pork Osso Buco, but I decided to switch to an easy comfort meal and make a pot roast since there were no pork butts with the bone in left at the market. I ended up with an incredibly simple pork roast with root veggies recipe that couldn't have turned out any better. So quick and delicious!

You'll start off preparing the vegetables. All you need to do is combine the carrots, celery, onion and garlic in a large bowl. Drizzle with olive oil and season with salt and pepper and set aside.

Preheat oven to 350º F. Pat the pork with paper towels until dry and lightly season with salt and pepper.

Put a Dutch oven over medium-high heat, then add 2 tbsp olive oil. When the oil is hot, add the roast and brown deeply on all sides, about 4 minutes per side.

Arrange potatoes, carrots, onion and garlic around pork. Add broth and toss to evenly coat vegetables.

Cover and place in lower portion of the oven. Roast 1 hour for boneless roast and 1 ¾ hours for bone-in roast. Halfway through roasting time, turn the roast over.

Transfer the roast to a cutting board. Spoon the vegetables and pan juices onto a large serving platter. Slice the roast, arrange the meat on top of the vegetables, and serve family style!

1 large (4 lbs) Boston pork butt

1 small bag (1 lb) California carrots, peeled

1 stalk of celery

4 Yukon gold potatoes

3 sweet onions

1 carton chicken broth

Extra virgin olive oil

Salt and pepper to taste

Serves 4–6

cara cara orange pineapple chicken

This is one of those recipes I made with ingredients I had available on-hand, so I didn't have to go to the market. I was running low on produce and had some fresh chicken that needed to be cooked—and quickly. Cara Cara oranges are navel oranges that are a bit like blood oranges. Their flesh is a ruby pink color. It only took one of these for this recipe, but they're a big part of what made this chicken so delicious! If you can't find a Cara Cara, then you can substitute a Navel orange instead.

Line a 13×9 casserole dish with extra virgin olive oil. Layer the bottom with one can of drained pineapple. Place the chicken on top of pineapple.

Slice the Cara Cara orange into wedges and place around the edges. The peel adds a nice fragrance and looks gorgeous.

Bake at 375º for one hour. Raise temp to 425º and keep a close eye on it until the top and edges are brown and crispy.

I served this with green beans but any veggies will work. If your house is stocked with fresh produce, then a mixed greens salad seems like the perfect accompaniment to this delicious dish!

1 package chicken thighs (approx. four bone-in, skin-on thighs)

1 package of chicken drumsticks (approx. 6 pieces)

1 can of pineapple, drained

1 Cara Cara orange, sliced

2 tablespoons extra virgin olive oil

Salt and pepper to taste

Serves 6—8

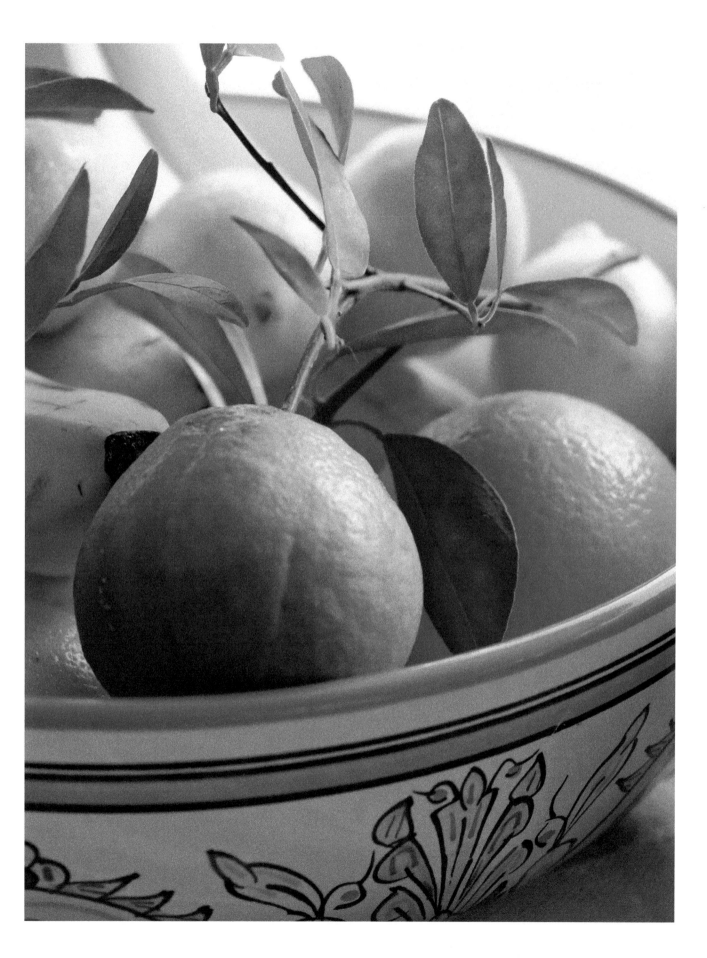

chicken thighs with broccoli slaw, asparagus and sweet onion

I use chicken thighs because dark meat has a better flavor. Plus, chicken thighs are hard to mess up. The ever present chicken breast will dry out quickly after cooking only a few minutes too long, but thighs are more forgiving. They can take the heat while staying juicy, tender and flavorful. It's kind of impossible to overcook them, which is why I love 'em. Keeping things simple in the kitchen is my M.O. for healthful eating and this simple and easy dinner only took 30 minutes to make!

Heat 1 tbsp. olive oil over medium-high heat in a cast iron skillet.

Sauté boneless, skinless chicken thighs about 6-7 minutes on one side, then turn over and add chopped onion to skillet. Cook an additional 6-7 minutes or until chicken is cooked through.

Remove chicken from skillet and add chopped asparagus and broccoli slaw. Sauté until the asparagus is bright green and crisp-tender, about 5-7 minutes.

Garnish with fresh or grilled peach slices and avocado to top off this healthy gluten free meal and make it summertime sweet!

½ bag broccoli slaw

1 package or bunch of asparagus, chopped

1 sweet onion, chopped

6 boneless, skinless chicken thighs

3 peaches, sliced

2 avocados, sliced

Extra virgin olive oil

Salt and pepper to taste

Serves 4–6

barbeque chicken with sweet onion, potatoes and spinach

This chicken is truly the BEST chicken recipe ever. I love making this dish for all my good friends that visit. The number one reason is because it's so simple. The second reason is because it's a comfort meal and everyone loves it. Easy doesn't have to mean out-of-the-can or frozen, nor does homespun have to mean unsophisticated or plain. My "fancy" meals are rather simple dishes so I know what I'm eating—and there's no gluten. So, grab your best ingredients and a bottle of vino and get ready for an impressive dinner without the fuss.

Preheat oven to 375º and line a 13×9 pan with enough olive oil to cover.

Place a layer of the chopped sweet onion over the olive oil, then the six boneless skinless chicken thighs on top. Bake about 40 minutes or until done, depending on your oven.

While the chicken is in the oven, cover a cast iron skillet with about 2 tbsp. of the olive oil. Add sliced potatoes and cook on medium heat until tender, adding more oil as needed to brown the potatoes.

In a separate pan or wok, heat 2 more tbsp. of the olive oil over medium heat. Add the spinach and cover for about 5 minutes. Stir in the garlic and cover again for another 5 minutes. Remove from heat.

Once the chicken is done, take the potatoes and sautéed spinach and interweave it into the chicken and bake another 5 minutes. You can top with whatever you like, but I love to stripe each thigh with barbeque sauce. Food art!

6 boneless, skinless chicken thighs

1 large sweet onion, chopped

6-8 cloves fresh garlic, minced

1 bag fresh spinach

3-4 medium Idaho or Russet potatoes, sliced

Extra virgin olive oil

Bone Suckin' Sauce, or your favorite gluten-free BBQ sauce

Serves 6

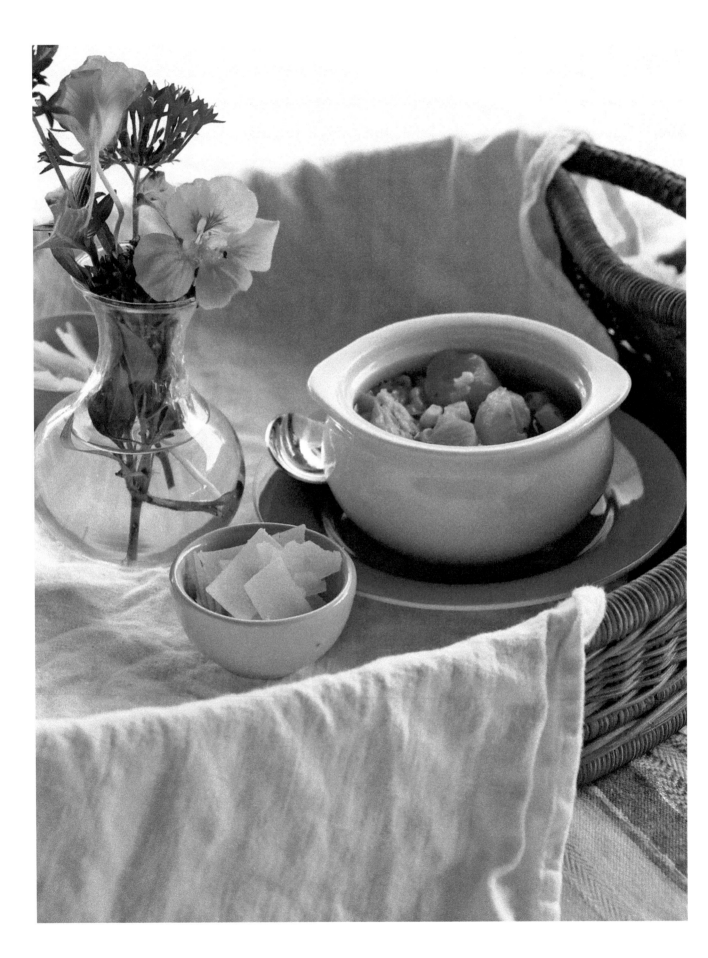

polenta chicken soup

You can make soup with just about anything in your kitchen and a little water. This polenta chicken soup is incredibly easy. Just add your own side salad and you've got yourself a satisfying, nutrient-filled and gluten-free meal. I made my salad with mixed greens, pecans, apples and bacon. Somehow it just came together with what we had in the fridge, but yours can be anything—your own special complementary creation!

In a large (approx. 5 quart) dutch oven or spaghetti pot, sautée chopped onion and chicken in a little bit of olive oil.

Add chopped carrots, celery, peas and corn, then fill dutch oven half full with water—covering ingredients. Simmer two hours. The chicken is usually so tender from the cooking process it just falls apart.

Right before you are ready to serve, slowly add ¼ cup of polenta, stirring with a wooden spoon until smooth and bubbly over medium heat. It thickens the soup and turns it into a meal.

Sprinkle with cheese and serve your choice of salad. If you're stuck on salad ideas, here are some of my favorite healthful, gluten-free treats to put on a bed of greens: garbanzo beans, corn, black beans, tomatoes, artichokes, dried cranberries, raisins and any variety of nuts.

If you keep these ingredients (and dressing) stocked in your fridge or pantry, you'll only need to remember to get the greens. You'll have magnificence, health and ease at your fingertips… or fork!

1 sweet onion

4 stalks celery

4 large peeled California carrots

4 boneless skinless chicken thighs

1 bag frozen sweet peas

1 cup frozen corn (optional)

¼ cup polenta

Extra virgin olive oil

Water

Parmesan cheese, grated (optional)

Salt and pepper to taste

Serves 4–6

groovy sunday sookie sookie soup

What do you do if you want some comfort food, but don't want any copycat version of a cookie? You queue up some Steppenwolf, turn up the volume and make my Sookie Sookie Soup! This is a great soup for a lazy Sunday and a healthy, satisfying meal that tantalizes your taste buds without compromising your wellness goals.

Chop the sweet onions and lightly sautée in a tiny bit of olive oil.

Place onions in the slow cooker and add the frozen sweet peas, fresh baby carrots, frozen lima beans and a handful of fresh cherry tomatoes. Once everything is in the crock pot add enough water to cover the veggies.

Turn the slow cooker on high heat and head-off for your afternoon hike. When you return, the house smells amazing and your craving for a cookie is long gone!

Top each bowl of Sookie with a few slices of avocado, 4-5 shrimp, and a sprinkle of parm.

2 sweet onions, chopped

1 bag (16 oz) baby carrots

1 bag (10-12 oz) frozen sweet peas

1 bag (10-12 oz) lima beans

Cherry tomatoes

Parsley, chili powder, cilantro, basil, or your choice of spice

Extra virgin olive oil

1 pound cooked shrimp, peeled and deveined

Avocado slices

Parmesan cheese, grated (optional)

Serves 6–8

veggie soup in the summertime

Hot soup in the summertime seems counterintuitive, but soup can be fun and comforting when the afternoon storms kick-up and you're indoors. Plus, staying hydrated is always important—especially when it's hot out. So, make your own homemade vegetable soup, tune into Shark Week on Discovery Channel and wait for the thunderstorms to stop!

Use your favorite soup pot or a 5-quart Dutch oven and fill with chopped celery, sweet onion and a tablespoon of olive oil. Sauté until soft.

Add the remaining veggies and and 5 cups of water.

Once soup has come to a boil, reduce to a simmer as the vegetables will overcook if your soup boils too vigorously.

Simmer for 30 minutes or until veggies are soft, but not mushy. Top with a sprinkle of shredded sharp cheddar cheese and salt and pepper, if desired.

4 sprigs fresh basil

1 small red onion

1 large sweet onion (or 2 small)

4 stalks of celery, chopped

2 zucchini, chopped

6 California carrots, peeled and chopped

½ head of cauliflower chopped

1 bag frozen organic spinach

1 cup frozen peas

5 cups water

Extra virgin olive oil

Serves 4–6

flounder with cello whisps

My Flounder with Cello Whisps recipe is incredibly fast and easy when you're looking for something light, lean, low-carb and gluten free—and don't want to spend a lot of prep time in the kitchen. Cello Whisps are Parmesan cheese crisps; a simple cracker, but with "real food" ingredients. They're made with baked parmesan cheese, that's it! Serve with a side of tartar sauce, lime and complementary veggie of your choice. Done!

On medium-high heat, sauté one sweet onion in a tablespoon of olive oil.

Add flounder fillets and let onions soften while cooking flounder evenly on both sides. It takes very little time to cook flounder because it's so thin. Be your own judge, depending on your pan and type of stove. I use a gas stove, so mine times out around 5 minutes.

Once the onions and flounder are about done, add 2 handfuls of fresh spinach and cook until wilted.

Place on a serving platter over cooked lima beans and add Cello Whisps to the top. You can use any brand of baked Parmesan cheese crisps, but these are my favorite.

Serve as-is or add sliced red bell peppers and avocado for added color, flavor and goodness!

1 small sweet onion

2 flounder fillets

1 tablespoon extra virgin olive oil

1 small bag of frozen lima beans

2 handfuls fresh spinach

1 lime

Cello Whisps (Parmesan crisps)

Tartar sauce (optional)

Serves 1–2

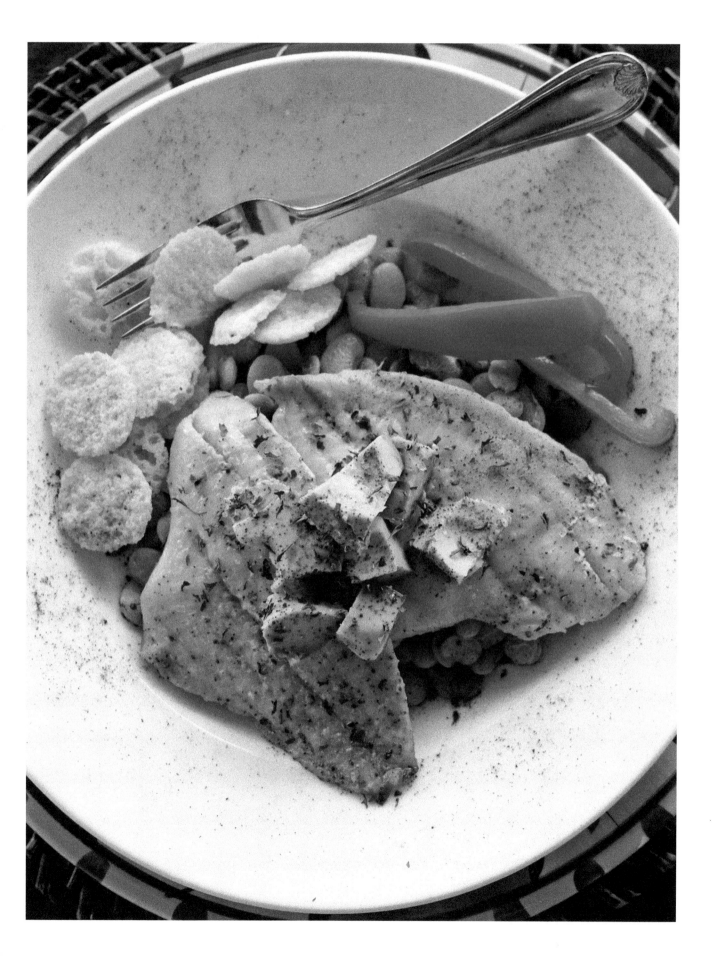

mussels (or clams) in white wine

Mussels are delicious, nutritious and quick and easy to make. They go great with pan-fried potatoes and a side salad. You can use the same recipe for clams, too (littlenecks, middlenecks, and topnecks—your choice). Be sure to cook them for a minimum of six minutes, discarding any clams that don't open within 10–15 min.

First, clean the mussels in cold, fresh water to remove any sand and grit before steaming them. Discard any mussels that are not tightly closed.

Saute 8 minced garlic cloves in olive oil in the bottom of a large sauce pan. Add parsley, oregano, basil and ¼ cup of cheese. Stir.

Add one cup of both water and wine to the olive oil and bring to a boil. Add mussels, stir well, reduce heat to medium and cover.

Steam mussels until they open. They cook rapidly (about 8–10 min) and are done when they open. Too much heat makes them dry and tough.

Place 6 on a plate, sprinkle with cheese and serve with a side of pan-fried potatoes to dip in the broth.

Pour the rest of slightly chilled white wine into glasses and serve!

_____

One 5 pound bag of Mussels

1 bottle of Pinot Grigio

8 garlic cloves

2 tablespoon olive oil

2 basil leaves

½ cup shaved aged Asiago cheese (optional)

A generous sprinkle of both parsley and oregano

_____

Serves 4

crab cake stuffed portobellos

I pulled out an old standby crab cakes recipe and painted my own gluten-free spin on an Old Bay® classic. I made these crab cakes by adding chopped sweet onions, yellow mustard and gluten-free bread crumbs in place of bread. I also did not use Worcestershire sauce or baking powder to keep 'em as clean as possible, but still crisp and golden on the outside.

Pour bread crumbs into large mixing bowl. I estimated around a half cup of gluten-free bread crumbs until it felt to be the right consistency. I usually use cornmeal in place of bread crumbs, but think bread crumbs work best for this recipe. (Gillian's Foods gluten-free bread crumbs are the best ones on the market with only rice flour, water, yeast, salt and cane sugar in their ingredients.)

Moisten with milk or coconut milk. Add mayonnaise, mustard and chopped onion; mix well. Add remaining ingredients and mix lightly.

Shape into 4 patties and refrigerate for 30 minutes to help keep the patties together when cooking. Broil or fry crab cakes until golden-brown on both sides.

Heat a grill or a large skillet over medium heat. Brush Portobello caps with olive oil to prevent sticking and cook on each side for 3-4 minutes, or until caramelized and deep golden brown.

To serve, place a crab cake on top of each of the Portobello caps alongside a green veggie or salad of your choice. I personally love sautéed fresh Brussels sprouts for a magnificently deeeelicious accompaniment and an elegant and simple dinner!

½ cup gluten-free bread crumbs or cornmeal

1 tablespoon mayonnaise

1 tablespoon yellow mustard

1 tablespoon parsley flakes

1 teaspoon Old Bay® seasoning

¼ teaspoon salt

1 egg beaten

Dash of milk (or coconut milk)

1 pound lump crab meat

½ of a medium sized sweet onion, chopped

4 Portobello mushroom caps, stems removed and wiped clean

Extra virgin olive oil

Serves 4

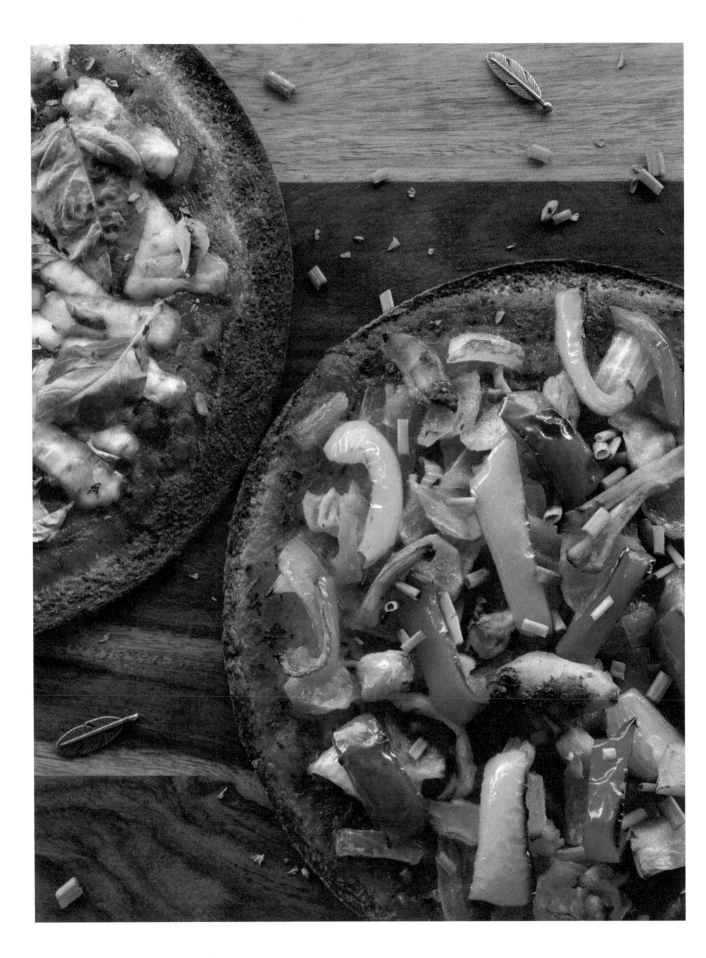

cauliflower crust pizza with bay scallops

I learned about Trader Joe's gluten-free cauliflower pizza crust from *Bon Appétit* magazine and tried it out after a family scalloping trip through Central Florida. This may be my new favorite hobby! It was like hunting and gathering; searching for buried treasure with the scallops shimmering in the sea grass. We traveled down the Econfina River from Econfina State Park out into the grassy flats of the Gulf. We collected our legal limit which made it possible to have them once at my sister-in-law's house and twice at mine!

Preheat the oven to 450°F. Pre-bake the gluten free cauliflower pizza crusts for approximately 10 minutes, then carefully flip and bake for another 10 minutes.

Drizzle enough olive oil to lightly coat bottom of cast iron skillet and add one tablespoon of salted butter. Sauté carrots, onion and pepper for 5 minutes at medium-high heat. Add tomatoes and cook an additional 2 minutes, then add spinach and sauté until wilted. Remove veggies from heat and set aside.

Rinse the scallops and pat dry with a paper towel. Sprinkle generously with salt and pepper.

Add 2 tsp olive oil and 1 tbsp butter to cast iron skillet and heat to medium-high. The pan needs to be very hot in order for the scallops to cook properly. You'll know the pan is hot enough if you drop some water on the pan and it evaporates instantly.

Place scallops in a single layer in skillet. You may need to cook them in several batches so you don't overcrowd the pan. Sauté scallops for 2 minutes, then flip and cook for another 2-3 minutes. If the scallops don't peel off the pan easily, let them cook for a few more seconds.

Top the pizza crusts with sautéed veggies and freshly grated parm. Place into the oven to warm at 400º until cheese is melted.

2 pre-made cauliflower pizza crusts (my favorite is Trader Joe's)

1 package of heavenly oval tomatoes, or your choice of grape tomatoes

2 California carrots, sliced

1 red pepper, diced

1 sweet onion, sliced

2 handfuls of fresh spinach

3 cups bay scallops

Extra virgin olive oil

1 tablespoon butter

¼ cup of white wine (I prefer a fruity and dry Pinot Grigio)

Freshly grated Parmesan cheese (optional)

Serves 4–6

shrimp cornbread muffins

If you have celiac disease or gluten intolerance, it's hard to find a cornbread mix without an added assortment of replacement flours. I also prefer a protein-packed muffin that's light on the carbs. My solution to both? These quick and easy, no flour, shrimp cornbread muffins! These muffins are tender and moist, and light on the sugar. While delicious just as it is, this cornbread recipe can also accommodate all kinds of personal touches like cheese, green onions, jalapeños, cilantro, lemon zest or any combo of your choice. Pair with a bowl of soup or salad, or serve as an hors d'oeuvre with an assortment of dipping sauces.

For the shrimp:

Heat about a tablespoon of coconut oil on medium high and add the garlic. Saute for a 20 seconds, then add shrimp. Cook for 3-4 minutes till the shrimp is cooked. Add a sprinkle of kosher salt.

For the muffins:

Combine eggs, cornmeal, buttermilk, baking powder, baking soda and salt in mixing bowl. Mix with large spoon or whisk.

Melt the coconut oil and pour it into the other ingredients, then mix.

Fill muffin cups about ¾ full, adding a shrimp to each one, then top with a sprinkle of paprika.

Bake until cornbread is springy in the middle and browned, about 15-20 minutes.

Although I love buttermilk anything, I've been dairy free since December 2017. Replacing dairy with almond milk is easy because there's no need to adjust the quantity. Make sure you get the plain almond milk for this recipe however, as it's sold in a variety of flavors and will alter the taste or color of your muffins.

---

12 shrimp, peeled and deveined

4 cloves of garlic

2 eggs

2 cups stone ground, whole grain cornmeal

2 cups buttermilk (or substitute almond milk)

1 teaspoon baking powder

1 teaspoon baking soda

¼ cup virgin coconut oil

½ teaspoon kosher salt

Paprika

12 paper cupcake wrappers

Serves 10-12

baked spaghetti squash

Baked spaghetti squash is a great replacement for pasta. It surpasses corn pasta or any gluten free pasta in how it tastes and makes you feel. It's light, delicious, full of vitamins and effortless to prepare. The BEST thing about spaghetti squash as a gluten-free alternative, is that once it's roasted, the fibrous, crunchy strands inside the squash can be scraped out to create long, thin "noodles." Spaghetti squash is incredibly versatile, easy to cook and has a mild taste, lending itself to all kinds of recipes. Keep in mind that even though it's called "spaghetti" squash, it does not taste like spaghetti.

Preheat oven to 375º. Cut a spaghetti squash in half. Remove the seeds and brush with olive oil. Season with salt and pepper to taste.

Place squash cut side down on a baking sheet and roast for 45–60 minutes or until tender. A good way to tell is if the cut sides are turning golden and the interiors are easily pierced through with a fork.

Remove squash from oven and turn cut side up to let cool for 10 minutes. Scrape out the spaghetti squash with a fork to remove spaghetti-like strands. If it seems hard to scrape out the insides, return to the oven for another 10 minutes. The squash should not be mushy, but have a nice, slight crunch—like pasta cooked al dente.

2 whole spaghetti squash

Extra virgin olive oil

Salt and pepper to taste

Serves 2–4

spaghetti squash boats with roasted butternut squash, brussels & shrimp

Instead of pasta, this recipe uses the roasted spaghetti squash, which shreds into thin, noodle-like strands when scraped with a fork after baking. I'm in love with spaghetti squash and think it's one of the BEST gluten-free spaghetti noodle substitutes out there. Plus, this recipe uses the self-made bowls that the noodles are already sitting in for super easy clean up. What's not to love about that?

Preheat oven to 375º. In a large bowl, combine the Brussels, butternut squash, olive oil, salt and pepper and arrange the vegetables on a baking sheet in a single layer. Bake 40 minutes, or until the veggies are tender.

Cut spaghetti squash in half lengthwise and scoop out the seeds. Drizzle with olive oil and season with a pinch of salt and pepper. Place cut side down on a baking sheet and bake alongside the butternut and brussels for 30 minutes.

While the veggies are in the oven, butterfly the shrimp by slicing down the vein line from the tail to the top. Slice as deep as possible without cutting all the way through. Season with salt and pepper and set aside.

To toast the crumbs, place desired amount in a large skillet and cook on medium heat. Keep an eye on the crumbs and toss until they start to brown. Lower the heat and stir the crumbs continually until toasted to your liking. Remove the crumbs immediately from the hot skillet.

Mix the eggs in a separate bowl and dip the shrimp in the egg mix to coat letting the excess drip off. Place on baking sheet, cut side down. Sprinkle bread crumbs over the top of the shrimp, then bake in the oven for 10-12 minutes.

Scrape the squash strands into a pile of "pasta" in the squash shells and top with the Brussels and butternut squash mixture and serve with a side of shrimp.

4-6 small spaghetti squash

1 butternut squash, peeled and cubed (or one 16 oz bag of frozen or fresh diced butternut squash)

1 bag (16 oz) Brussels sprouts, halved

1 pound large shrimp (21-25 count), peeled and deveined

2 large eggs

Extra virgin olive oil

Gillian's gluten-free bread crumbs, skillet toasted if desired

Parmesan cheese (optional)

Salt and pepper to taste

Serves 4—6

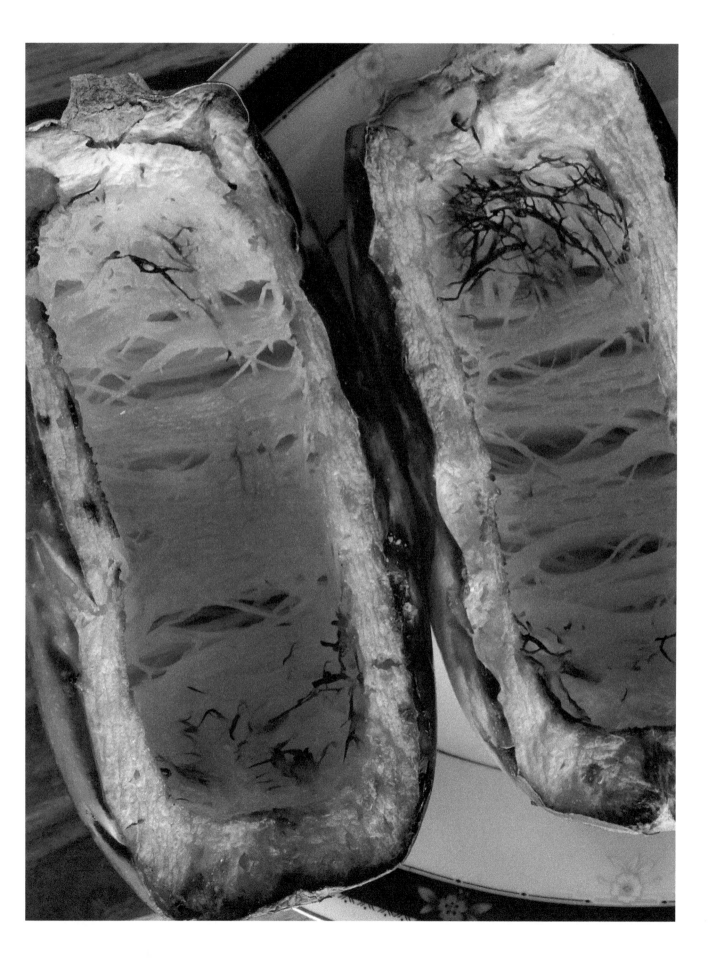

momma annabelle's chicken parmesan

I grew up with my 100% Italian mom and grandma making stuffed shells or homemade manicotti for Christmas. I made those for my boys and husband every December until I had to switch to a gluten-free diet. To stick close to our Italian family tradition, I now make a gluten-free chicken Parmesan that my mom Annabelle taught me how to make. I used my favorite sauce, Rao's Marinara, for this recipe. However, Annabelle would never use a pre-made sauce like Rao's. She makes her own, which I do on occasion. But sometimes convenience trumps gourmet, and that's when a trusty jar of marinara sauce can save the day!

Mix together 2 cups of Gillian's bread crumbs, 1 cup of grated Parmesan cheese and a sprinkle of both parsley and basil in a shallow dish.

In a separate bowl, mix together both eggs and a dash of milk. Add chicken until moist.

Place olive oil on the bottom of 9×13 Pyrex glass baking dish. Dredge each cutlet in the bread crumb and Parmesan cheese mixture and place cutlets evenly in pan with an additional sprinkle of olive oil on top. Bake at 350º for 30 minutes.

When done, remove from oven and add a topping of Rao's sauce to each cutlet and a slice of fresh buffalo mozzerella. Put back in oven until melted.

Add any twist to make it your own: mushrooms, more cheese, less cheese, etc. I like to add oven roasted zucchini slices and brussels sprouts for color and an extra serving of veggies!

One jar (16 oz) of Rao's Marinara

6 chicken cutlets

2 eggs

2 cups of Gillian's gluten-free bread crumbs

Grated Parmesan cheese

Fresh parsley and basil

1 package (8 oz) buffalo mozzarella (optional)

Milk or almond milk

Salt and pepper to taste

Serves 4–6

jet's marinara sauce and zoodles

This delicious dinner will give you zoodles of energy, and trading high-carb pasta for veggies is a great way to eat, whether you have celiac or not. Spiralized veggie noodles are my new favorite thing. I've been spiralizing zucchini for a while as an alternative to pasta, but these fun, twisted vegetables seem to be everywhere; along with so many great recipes and ideas for easy gluten-free meals. Spiralized veggie noodles are a cinch to make. But if you don't have a spiralizer or are on-the-go, then you can buy them pre-made. Veggie Noodle Co. has a great variety to choose from, too: zucchini, beet, sweet potato and butternut squash.

For the sauce:

In a large sauce pan or spaghetti pot, drizzle in the olive oil, then sauté a garlic clove or one inch of garlic paste. Don't let it get too hot.

Add in one can of tomato paste and one can equal parts water. Stir. Add the peeled tomatoes. I used a potato masher to break them up. It makes the sauce thicker and richer. Add the bay leaf and spices to taste.

Simmer on low for at least an hour. Momma Annabelle simmers hers for two. Of course the ultimate yummy thing is to add meatballs, but pre-cook the meatballs until almost done, then let them cook the rest of the way in the sauce. You could also add onion, mushrooms and Italian sausage that you pre-cook.

For the zoodles:

For the zoodles, you'll need a spiralizer (or julienne peeler). Just follow the instructions for your spiralizer in the insert. There's really no prepping or cooking of any kind. You could easily stir-fry your zoodles or place them in a microwave-safe dish and cook on high for 2 minutes if you prefer them warm, but not soggy. Zucchini is a high water content vegetable, so the longer zucchini cooks, the more water is released and the more mushy it gets.

1 can (6 oz) tomato paste

1 can (28 oz) of Italian peeled tomatoes in tomato purée

Garlic or garlic paste

2 tablespoons extra virgin olive oil

Chopped parsley and oregano

1 bay leaf

6 zucchini

Freshly ground pepper

Serves 2–4

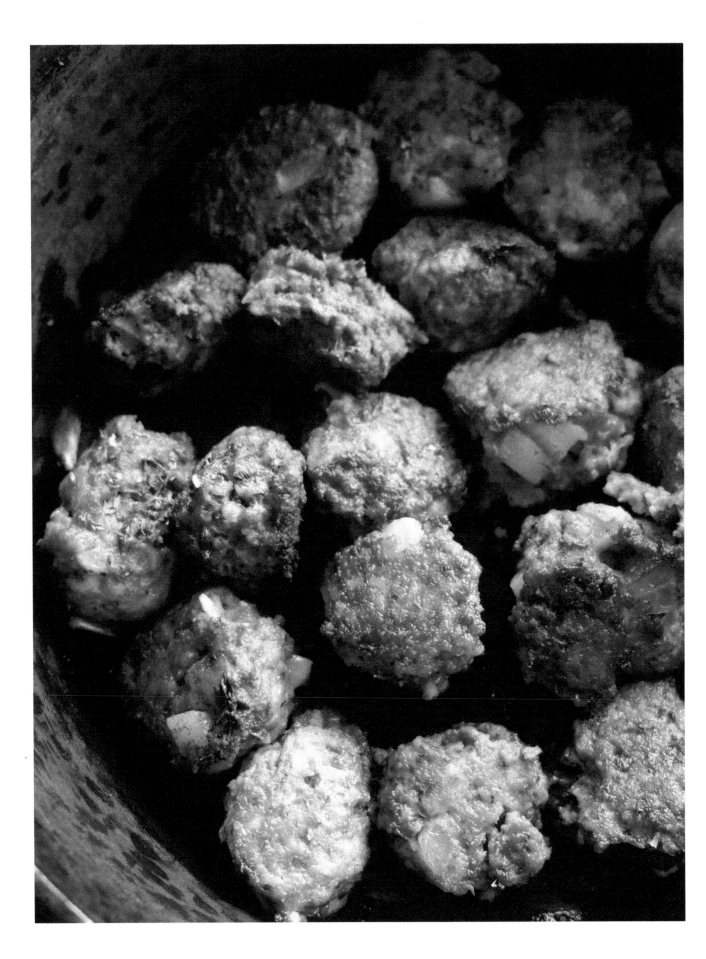

rustic italian meatballs

Meatballs are a superpower food for me and a simple way to please a room full of hungry eaters. I love to experiment with them in a variety of tasty ways with an emphasis on healthy, gluten-free, low-carb and easy. You can change up the meat, vary the seasonings, add extra ingredients and even cook the meatballs in different ways. I have many meatball recipes to share, and this one is my take on an old Italian favorite.

In a large mixing bowl, combine the ground chuck with the onion, garlic and spinach using hands. Crack the egg into the bowl and mix it into the ground chuck mixture. You don't want to over-mix the meatballs and the light touch of your hands combines the ingredients without crushing the meat.

Add the Parmesan cheese, spices and breadcrumbs to the mixture and knead until well combined. Full pieces of ground meat should still be visible. Form the mixture into meatballs approximately 1 ½ inches in size.

Heat the olive oil over medium heat and add the meatballs to the pan. Cook for 15-20 minutes, rolling them around frequently to ensure even browning.

Remove the meatballs and place them into a baking dish. Pour enough marinara sauce over the meatballs and sprinkle with shredded mozzarella.

Bake at 375º for 10 minutes, or until cheese is melted and browned. Serve!

1 small sweet onion, chopped

1 ½ pounds ground chuck

1 egg

1 cup Gillian's gluten-free bread crumbs

1 cup Parmesan cheese (optional)

1 teaspoon each dried basil, oregano and parsley flakes

1 teaspoon garlic, minced

1 handful fresh spinach

1 jar (24 oz) Rao's Marinara sauce

2 tablespoons extra virgin olive oil

1 cup shredded mozzarella cheese (optional)

Salt and pepper to taste

Serves 4–6

marry me meatballs

Sometimes, you just feel it in your bones: This is the one for me. And when that happens, you make up your mind, no reservations. The reason these are called "Marry Me" meatballs is because the moment you take one bite of these, you'll be swept off your feet. There's a cube of mozzarella in the center of each meatball —perfectly melted. Consider yourself committed!

In a large mixing bowl, combine the ground turkey with the onion, zucchini and parsley, using hands. Crack the egg into the bowl and knead it into the ground turkey mixture.

Add the Parmesan cheese and cornmeal to the mixture and knead until well combined.

Form the mixture into meatballs adding a cube of mozzarella to the center of each one.

Heat olive oil over medium heat with a tablespoon of butter for a nice, crispy outside.

Place meatballs in pan, turning each until all sides are golden brown. Lower heat and cover them to cook. Make sure cooked all the way through, about 20 minutes.

Add marinara sauce and simmer for 10 more minutes. Sprinkle a tiny bit of shredded Parm over the top to taste.

¼ cup cornmeal (a yummy and healthy alternative to bread crumbs!)

¼ cup grated Parmesan cheese

1 egg

1 ¼ pounds ground turkey (or ground chuck)

1 sweet onion, chopped

1 small zucchini, chopped

2 teaspoons dried parsley

1 tablespoon extra virgin olive oil

1 tablespoon butter

1 package (8 oz) mozzarella, cubed

1 jar (24 oz) Rao's Marinara

Salt and pepper to taste

Serves 4—6

aussie bbq meatballs

These BBQ meatballs are one of those fun foods that double as an appetizer or a main dish. The first time I had Aussie anything was similar to these meatballs, but in a burger. You can do the same with a gluten-free bun for a hero or hoagie sandwich. I eat them plain and love 'em that way, but you can serve over rice with and top with peas as an easy, yummy option!

In a large bowl mix together the ground chuck, cornmeal, mayo, parsley, gluten-free teriyaki sauce and a sprinkle of chili powder, using hands.

Crack the egg into the bowl and knead it into the ground chuck mixture. Form into meatballs.

Add just enough olive oil to cover bottom of sauté pan and cook meatballs on medium heat.

In a separate grill pan, grill pineapple rings with a splash of teriyaki sauce until bubbly and grill marks appear. Add orange slices.

In a separate sauce pan, mix the pineapple juice from the can with two teaspoons of corn starch on medium heat until thickened. Pour sauce over finished meatballs and serve on their own, or top with green peas over rice!

1 ¼ pounds ground chuck

1 can (20 oz) pineapple rings

4 tablespoons gluten-free teriyaki sauce

1 cup cornmeal or gluten-free bread crumbs

1 egg

½ cup mayonnaise

1 Naval orange, sliced

2 teaspoons corn starch

1 teaspoon parsley

Sprinkle of chili powder

Salt and pepper to taste

Serves 4–6

cowboy meatballs

I love this recipe because it combines two of my favorites: meatballs and Mexican food. I love to eat Mexican food at home and especially when I travel; mostly because it's easy to find gluten-free choices. Serve these up with a big bowl of guacamole and any of your favorite salsas. There are additional toppings you can add too, like cilantro, shredded cabbage or lettuce, and asadero cheese for a more authentic Mexican taste.

In a large bowl mix together: ground pork, minced garlic, cornmeal (or bread crumbs) and 1 can of refried black beans, using hands.

Crack the eggs into the bowl and knead it into the ground pork mixture. Form into small-sized meatballs so they cook through faster and fit inside the taco shells.

Add just enough olive oil to cover bottom of sauté pan and add meatballs. Cook on medium heat until browned and cooked through.

Add salsa of your choice to pan (optional).

In a separate pan on medium heat, saute red peppers and sweet onions until soft.

Turn oven to 375º to warm up the taco shells for a couple of minutes. Place meatballs in warm shells and top the way you like it!

---

1 package blue corn taco shells

2 red peppers

1 sweet onion

Extra virgin olive oil

1 ¼ pounds ground pork

½ teaspoon minced garlic

2 eggs

1 jar (16 oz) of your favorite salsa

½ cup cornmeal or gluten-free bread crumbs

1 can Amy's refried black beans (or another brand that you know is gluten-free)

Serves 4–6

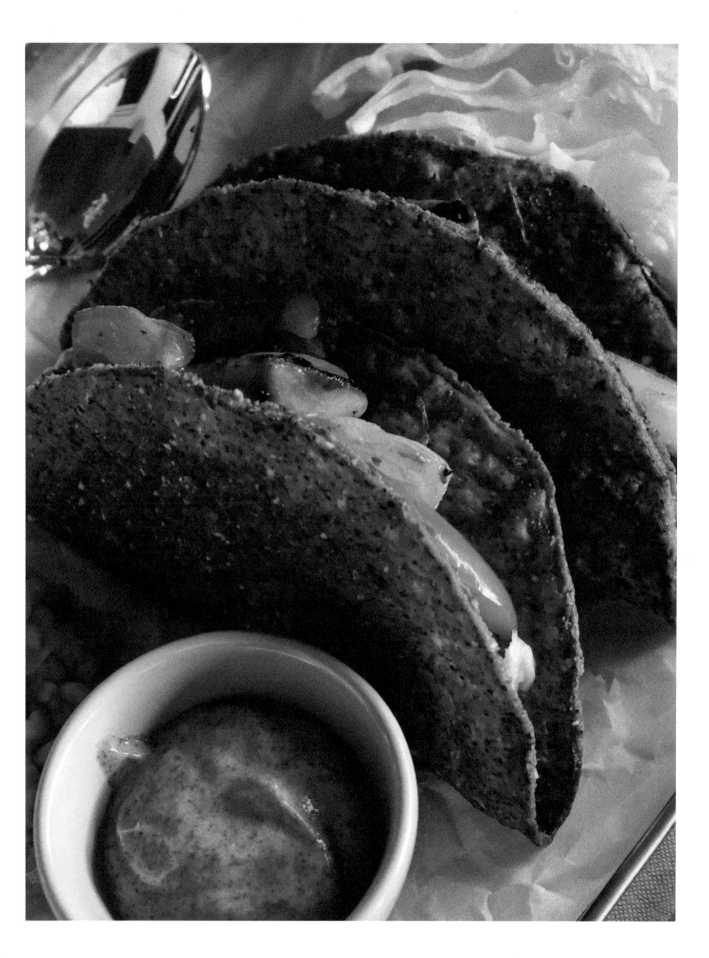

simple one-skillet lettuce wraps

You probably don't associate "light" cooking with a cast iron skillet, as usually what comes to mind are meals like cheesy casseroles and cornbread pies. But I love my Lodge cast-iron skillet! It's incredibly versatile and cooks food evenly with a beautiful outer crust. I like to freestyle in the kitchen and this simple, one-skillet meal keeps things easy breezy and makes a large quantity, so it's great if you're having guests over.

Warm the skillet and olive oil over medium to medium-high heat and add the ground chuck to the center of the pan. I get my beef from the butcher or Fresh Market, as they grind it on the premises and it's completely yummy and fresh, not from a package.

Use a stiff spatula or wooden spoon to break the ground chuck into smaller pieces. Sprinkle with salt and minced garlic and stir the beef occasionally to make sure it's browning evenly. The beef is finished when it's evenly browned and shows no signs of pink.

Reduce heat to low and add spinach and cherry tomatoes. Stir until well combined.

Scoop the meat and veggie mixture onto your favorite lettuce leaves. I use butterhead lettuce for its flavor and texture as it works well as a wrapper for foods.

1 pound ground chuck

½ teaspoon of garlic, minced

1 container (8 oz) cherry tomatoes

1 bag of fresh baby spinach

1 tablespoon extra virgin olive oil

1 head butter, bibb or iceburg lettuce

Salt and pepper to taste

Serves 6–8

spaghetti squash tacos

Maybe you like spaghetti squash as a vegetable, but don't love it as a substitute for good ol' pasta. That's okay! I've got another easy and delicious way you can add this healthy veggie to your diet. These tacos are great as-is without anything else on top, though avocados would make a nice touch. But honestly, I love the pure and simple and these spaghetti squash tacos won my heart for easy and pleasing!

Preheat oven to 375º. Cut spaghetti squash in half lengthwise and scoop out the seeds. Drizzle with olive oil and season with a pinch of salt and pepper. Place cut side down on a baking sheet and bake for 45 minutes or until tender.

While spaghetti squash is baking, lightly coat a large skillet with olive oil and sauté ground chuck until browned, breaking it into smaller pieces as it cooks. Set aside.

When spaghetti squash is done, add the "noodles," spinach, salt, pepper and cherry tomatoes. Sauté on low heat for about 5–8 more minutes.

Serve in corn tortillas or taco shells with your toppings of choice: cilantro, chopped green onion, jalapenos, guacamole, salsa, sour cream or shredded cheese all work great!

1 package corn tortillas or blue corn taco shells (8–10 count)

1 ½ pounds ground chuck

½ of a baked spaghetti squash

½ bag of chopped spinach

1 container (8 oz) cherry tomatoes

Extra virgin olive oil

Salt and pepper to taste

Serves 6–8

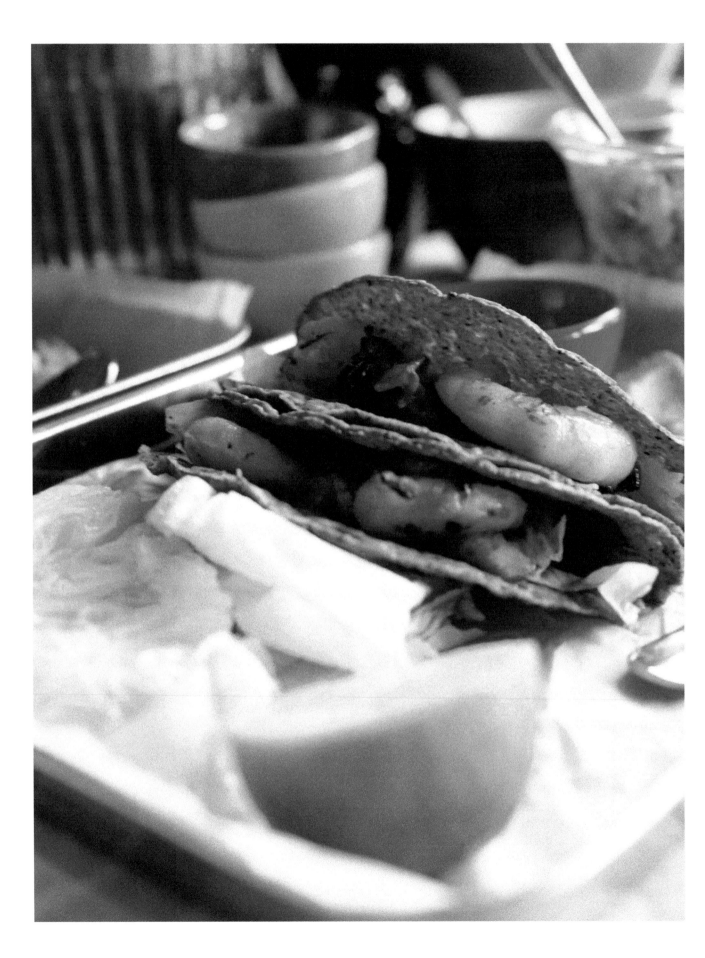

shrimp tacos with chili-lime mayo

In addition to being healthy, shrimp cooks in a matter of minutes, making it ideal for my kind of "fast food." The trick to getting the shrimp perfectly cooked is by heating your skillet until it's very hot. I like to use my Lodge cast-iron for this because it retains the heat, but any heavy-duty skillet will work well.

For the chili-lime mayo:

Squeeze half of the fresh lime into the mayo. Sprinkle in ½ teaspoon minced garlic and chili powder to taste. Place in fridge.

For the shrimp tacos:

Warm the skillet over medium-high heat for approx. 2 minutes or until it's very hot. Add shrimp, olive oil and 1 teaspoon minched garlic and sauté until pink. Set aside.

Warm corn tortillas in a skillet or taco shells in the oven for a few minutes. Place cooked shrimp and cabbage mixture in warm tortillas and add chili lime mayo and sliced avocado to top!

1 package corn tortillas or blue corn taco shells (8–10 count)

1 pound large shrimp (21-25 count), peeled with tails off

Extra virgin olive oil

1 cup mayonnaise

1 lime

Chili powder

1 ½ teaspoons garlic, minced

1 prebagged shredded cabbage, broccoli, kale, and Brussels sprouts mixture (or shredded lettuce of your choice)

1 Hass avocado

Serves 6–8

twice as nice pinwheel salad

I'm a big fan of leftovers and ground beef is one of the most versatile ingredients around. This quick and easy salad is made with leftover burgers, salsa and blue cheese* dressing, but you can also try it with turkey, chicken, lamb or pork. I think the Pinwheel Salad is delicious by itself, but you can change it up by adding a different salad dressing, corn, black beans or tomatoes. It all sounds great to me!

Line your plate with tortilla chips and shredded sweet butter lettuce in the center.

Slice some avocados and place on top, then add salsa of your choice.

Crumble burgers and reheat. Sprinkle on top of your salad and add blue cheese, ranch or cilantro-lime dressing.

*Just to be safe, you may want to stay away from all "moldy" or ripened cheeses like blue cheese to avoid potential gluten, as some sources suggest that mold cultures of cheese may be grown on wheat or rye bread. I've never had any complications from eating blue cheese, but recommend that you *always* read the ingredients label carefully and contact the manufacturer for questions about specific products, if you are unsure.

Sweet butter lettuce

Sliced avocado

Salsa

Tortilla chips

Blue cheese, ranch or cilantro-lime dressing*

Leftover ground chuck angus burgers

Serves 2–4

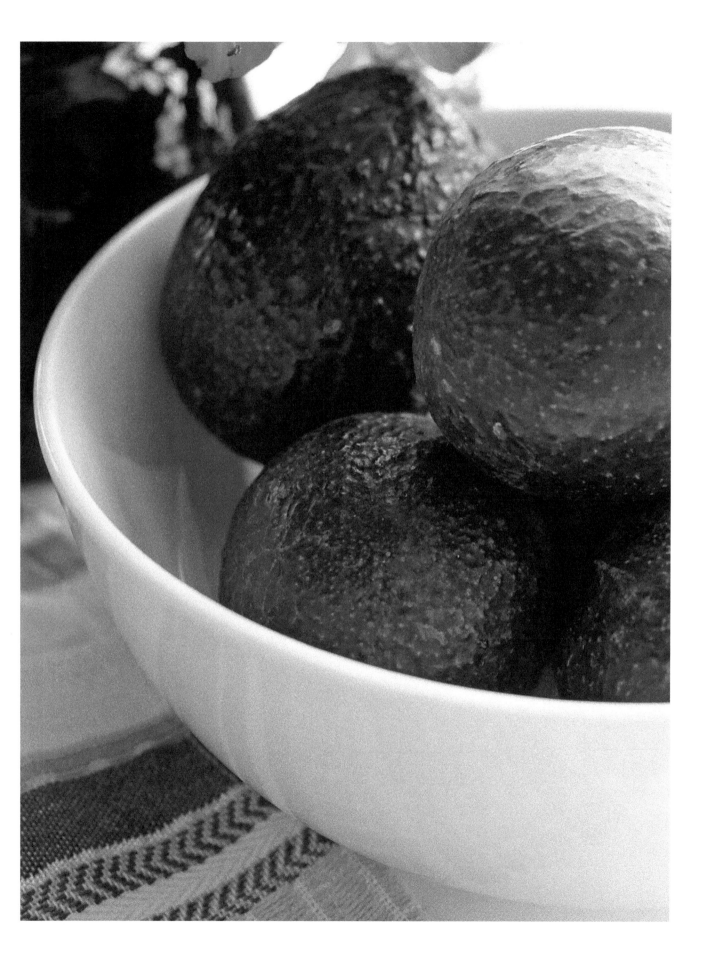

salad is fresh and light
meatballs are hardy
put them together
now there's a delicious party!

– jet –

caesar salad with meatballs, asparagus and portobellos

You can't eat meatballs without a salad. It's just not right! And in the summertime, how 'bout meatballs on top of your romaine lettuce instead of croutons? We don't want to overload simple meals with too many things, but there's always a way to make anything healthier... and that is to add veggies! I topped this with some asparagus and portobello mushrooms with melted provolone for a unique, delicious, gluten-free Caesar salad.

For the meatballs:

In a large mixing bowl, combine the ground chuck with the ground pork, using hands. Crack the eggs into the bowl and add bread crumbs or cornmeal to the mixture and knead until well combined. Form the mixture into meatballs.

Add 2 tablespoons olive oil to sauté pan on medium-high heat, then add a tablespoon of butter if you would like to get a nice crispy outside. Place meatballs in pan, turning each until all sides are golden brown. Lower heat to medium and cook all the way through—about 20 min.

Add your favorite marinara sauce and simmer for 10 more minutes, or until slightly bubbly. Sprinkle with shredded Parm to taste.

For the portobellos and asparagus:

Drizzle 3 tablespoons of olive oil over both sides of the mushrooms. Sprinkle with salt and pepper. Cook on a stove-top griddle or grill pan until the mushrooms are heated through and tender, about 5 minutes per side. Top with sliced provolone.

Heat 1 tbsp. olive oil or butter in a large skillet over medium-high heat. Add asparagus spears. Cover and cook for 10 minutes, stirring occasionally, until asparagus is tender.

For the caesar salad:

Place the lettuce in a large bowl. Cut portobellos into quarters. Top with asparagus slices and portobello mushrooms. Sprinkle with red pepper flakes. Top with meatballs and your favorite GF Caesar salad dressing.

---

2 pounds ground chuck/ground pork mixture (1 ¼ chuck, ¾ pork)

1 cup Gillian's gluten-free breadcrumbs or cornmeal

2 eggs

Extra virgin olive oil

Butter

Marinara Sauce

Parmesan cheese

1 bunch medium-size asparagus stalks

7 large portobello mushrooms (about 5 inches in diameter), stemmed

Provolone cheese slices

1 large head romaine lettuce, cleaned and cut into large pieces (about 1-2 inches)

Red pepper flakes

Gluten-free Caesar salad dressing

Salt and pepper to taste

Serves 6–8

sweet corn and watermelon salad

This beautiful and delicious summer salad contains seasonal veggies, fruits and herbs that I'm positively positive will leave you feeling well and optimally optimistic! Because my diet is an 80/20 blend of single ingredient whole foods, I love eating and meal planning according to the seasons. I've found that it's the most simple, delicious and stress-free way to maintain a gluten-free lifestyle around celiac disease.

For the dressing:

In a small bowl, whisk olive oil, lime juice, salt and pepper. Set aside.

For the salad:

In a large skillet, cook and stir corn over medium-high heat until tender. Transfer to a salad bowl to cool.

Divide lettuce onto four plates. Top each portion with watermelon, corn, mint and cheese, dividing evenly. Drizzle with dressing over all.

_____

One head of butter, bibb or iceberg lettuce

2 cups diced watermelon

1 ½ cups sweet corn kernels

2 tablespoons mint, chopped

¼ cup crumbled feta cheese (optional)

2 tablespoons extra virgin olive oil

1 tablespoon lime juice

Salt and pepper to taste

_____

Serves 4

strawberry spring mix with flaked crab

What makes a regular salad a summer salad? Shoot, anything in season. These include hydrating fruits and vegetables like fresh corn, watermelon, cucumber, zucchini, tomatoes, strawberries, grapes... the list goes on. Simply add to a bowl of big leafy greens and you've nailed it! Add lean, healthy proteins to power up your salads with little-to-no preparation like this flaked crab, and easily transform it into a filling meal that will keep you satisfied.

Hull and slice each strawberry into 6 pieces if you have large strawberries and 4 pieces if strawberries are small.

Divide spring mix onto four plates. Break up the crab meat slightly, if jumbo lump crab meat.

Top each spring mix portion with crab meat and strawberries, dividing evenly. Squeeze fresh lemon juice over the top and add salt and pepper to taste.

*I like to use fresh crab meat as much as possible, however keeping things stocked and simple in the kitchen keeps me on track. You can find Phillip's jumbo lump crab meat in the freezer aisle of most grocery stores, as well as a frozen version made by Trader Joe's.

1 bag spring mix

1 package (8 oz) fully cooked wild caught crab meat*

10 fresh strawberries

Freshly squeezed lemon juice

Salt and pepper to taste

Serves 4

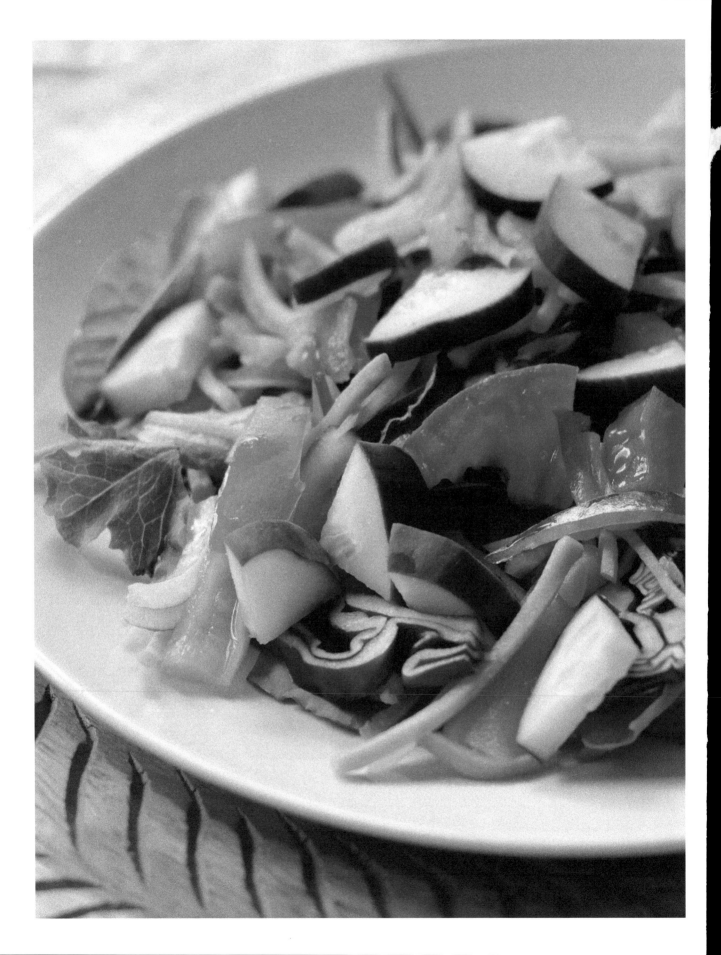

everything in the fridge salad

My general mealtime rule of thumb is there must be something green on the plate, and oftentimes this means salad! I love to experiment and incorporate seasonal fruits and vegetables into my salads in all colors of the rainbow. A bag of romaine hearts, shredded carrots and pre-shredded cabbage, along with a jar of roasted red peppers and a red onion from the pantry, are all delicious veggies that make for a good base and will keep in the fridge for a while without spoiling. Having these healthy basics on hand make for easy meal prep for grab-and-go salads all week!

Cut or tear romaine leaves into bite-size pieces. Divide lettuce onto individual serving plates.

Cut or julienne onion into thin slices. Add equal portions of shredded carrots, cabbage and roasted peppers, and top with a vinaigrette dressing of your choice. I think the best ones have just the right touch of sweetness, but not a lot of sugar. Check the labels and look for ones with 3 grams or less.

This recipe makes for a good base, but the sky's the limit for salad toppings. Lean protein choices like string cheese, canned chickpeas, nuts and cubed or sliced meats are a great addition, as well as other fresh veggie items you have on hand like a handful of spring mix, cucumbers and tomatoes—whatever your heart desires!

1 bag romaine hearts

1 bag pre-shredded carrots

1 bag pre-shredded red cabbage

1 jar roasted pepper slices

Red onion, sliced

Garlic Expressions classic vinaigrette salad dressing, or gluten-free vinaigrette dressing of your choice

Serves 4–6

italian roasted veggies

This mixture of veggies is such a simple, easy, delicious and gluten-free way to roast up some vegetables Italian style. I chose a combination of roasted cauliflower, mushrooms and cherry tomatoes, and served with a side of broccoli slaw marinara. This makes a hearty sauce with no pasta needed. You can place the sauce on top of your roasted veggies, or on the side, and add grated Parmesan to top.

For the roasted veggies:

Preheat oven to 375º. Cover a large cookie sheet with a light sprinkle of olive oil, then add sliced cauliflower, mushrooms and cherry tomatoes.

Sprinkle top of veggies with an additional 1-2 tablespoons olive oil and add a pinch of equal parts parsley, red pepper and basil. Bake for 30 minutes.

For the broccoli slaw marinara:

While vegetables are roasting, lightly coat a large skillet with olive oil and turn heat to medium.

Add marinara sauce and one package of broccoli slaw and cook until heated through and broccoli slaw is tender.

---

1 head cauliflower, chopped

1 package (16 oz) of sliced button mushrooms

1 medium-sized carton or clamshell of cherry tomatoes

Extra virgin olive oil

Red pepper

Fresh parsley and basil (dried will work too, if you don't have any available)

1 jar (24 oz) of your favorite—or homemade—marinara sauce

1 package broccoli slaw

Parmesan cheese, grated

Serves 4–6

artichoke hearts with bacon parm crisp

A favorite high-fiber veggie of mine is the artichoke. The beautiful thing about artichokes is that they can be a meal in and of themselves. Many people love artichokes, but don't prepare them at home. I agree that their thorny exterior is intimidating, but they have so many nutrients in that big heart! I've read recipes on how to prepare and cook them on the stovetop, but I used a box of frozen artichoke hearts to save time and keep it simple.

Line bottom of an 8 x 8 Pyrex casserole dish with olive oil. Place frozen artichokes in a single layer and sprinkle with chopped sweet onions.

Layer breadcrumbs or cornmeal on top of the artichokes, then Parmesan, then a layer of bacon. Drizzle with melted butter. The little bit of butter gives it the toasted brown color.

Bake at 375º for 30 minutes or until golden brown and onions are tender.

---

1 box (9 oz) frozen artichoke hearts

1 sweet onion, chopped

½ cup bacon pieces

½ cup parmesan cheese, grated (optional)

½ cup Gillian's gluten-free bread crumbs or cornmeal

1 tablespoon butter, melted (optional)

Extra virgin olive oil

Serves 4–6

campfire potatoes and sweet onions

If you love camping and love breakfast, then you're going to love this! It's enough for a small army, so wait til your kids come home and bring their friends and make a breakfast feast. You can adjust the amounts to feed your crew, you… or just two! I love to treat myself with a super satisfying, calorie-dense meal before hitting the trails. Campfire it up on the road or at home. You don't have to wait for a camping trip to make s'mores, eat a big ol' watermelon out on the porch or make these kick-ass potatoes and onions.

Line the bottom of a cast-iron skillet with coconut oil and place over medium-high heat.

When oil responds to one slice of potato, place the rest in the skillet in a single layer. Add onions. Flip and cook until golden brown.

Serve with a side of bacon and eggs for camping, or glam 'em up for Sunday brunch under a delicious gluten-free Eggs Benny topped with bacon, perfectly poached eggs and a creamy hollandaise sauce. Breakfast for everyone!

5 Idaho potatoes, sliced

2 sweet onions, sliced

1 tablespoon extra virgin coconut oil or avocado oil

Salt and pepper to taste

Serves 6–8

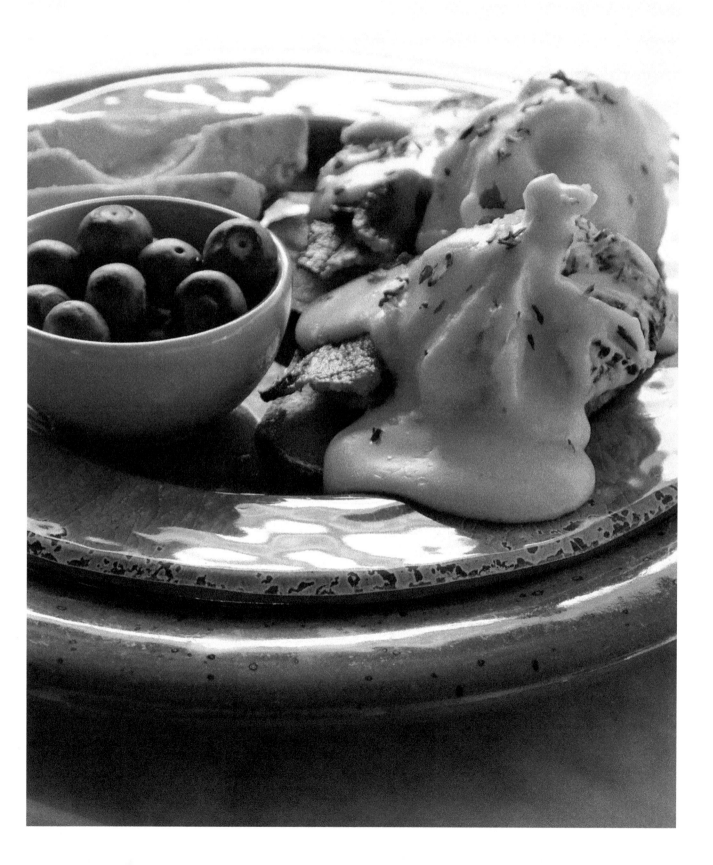

stovetop frittata for four

A frittata is basically an Italian omelet, or a quiche without the crust. There are two ways to cook a frittata: Either on the stove or baked in the oven. I prefer the stove-top version since it's the quickest and easiest way. I tend to use whatever I have on hand for omelets or frittatas, and came up with this using leftover veggies from a weekend cookout. I did not use ricotta cheese–which is common for frittatas—but substituted cheddar for all the cheese lovers in my family.

Coat the bottom of a skillet with olive oil, or a combination of 1 tablespoon olive oil and 1 tablespoon butter. Heat on medium-high heat until the oil is shimmering, then add sliced mushrooms, peppers and onions.

While the veggies are cooking, whisk together the eggs in a small bowl with a splash of water.

Cook mushrooms, peppers and onions until caramelized, then set aside. Reduce heat to medium. Add the eggs and cook for 2-3 minutes stirring constantly, until the eggs begin to scramble. Add broccoli slaw. Stop stirring and allow the eggs to continue cooking until they set.

Top with shredded cheddar and season with salt and pepper to taste.

½ cup button mushrooms (sliced and sauteed)

½ cup sweet union (sliced and sauteed)

1 handful broccoli slaw

4 eggs

½ cup sharp cheddar cheese, shredded (optional)

Extra virgin live oil

Butter (optional)

Salt and pepper to taste

Serves 4

how we roll breakfast casserole

Loaded with a healthy head o' broccoli, this simple gluten-free breakfast casserole is perfect for holiday brunches or make-ahead family breakfasts. And unlike many egg casserole recipes, this one substitutes shredded hash browned potatoes for bread. You can make it the night before if you're short on time in the mornings, or have a full house for the holidays. Serve with fresh fruit to keep it satisfying without weighing you down. Breakfast is how we roll!

Preheat oven to 375º. While oven is pre-heating, chop broccoli into small florets. Set aside.

Heat a cast-iron or heavy skillet to medium-high heat and sauté hash browned potatoes in coconut oil until golden brown. I used half the bag to keep it low-carb, but you can add more potatoes. It's your preference!

Line a 13 x 9 casserole dish with cooked potatoes and place provolone slices on top to cover the potatoes.

Scramble six eggs with a splash of milk and pour over the top. Sprinkle chopped broccoli over the egg mixture. Bake for 30 minutes until golden brown.

---

1 head of fresh broccoli, chopped

6 eggs

Splash of milk or almond milk

1 tablespoon extra virgin coconut oil or avocado oil

½ bag of Alexia Yukon Select shredded hash browns

6 slices of provolone cheese (optional)

Serves 6–8

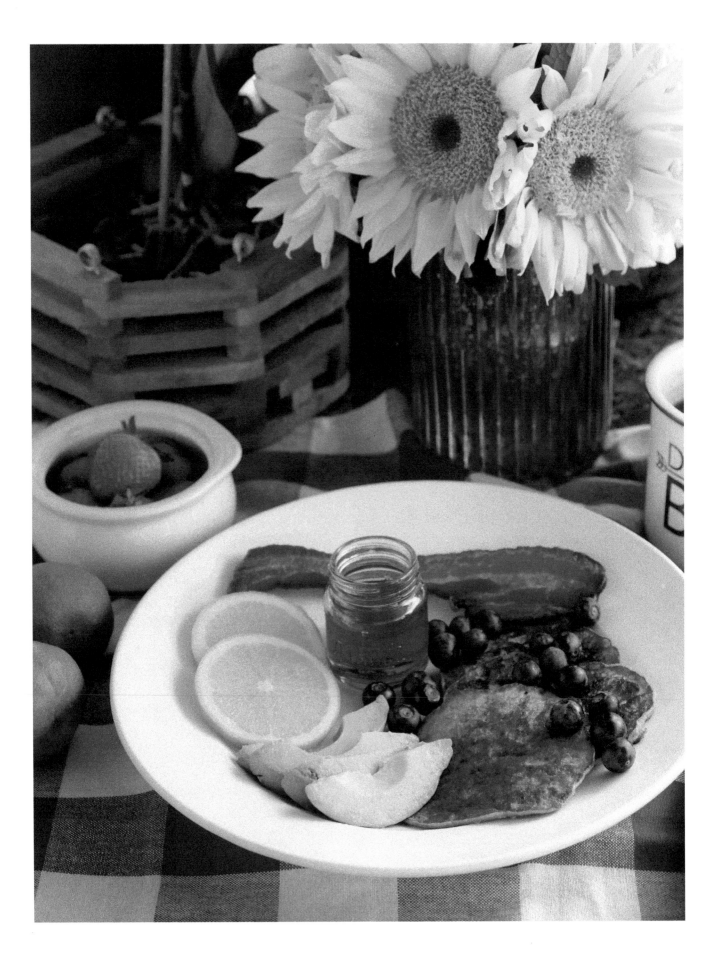

no flour banana pancakes

These ain't yo' momma's pancakes and you won't find 'em at IHOP. Most of us grew up with Bisquick or Betty Crocker pancakes made with Gold Medal All Purpose Flour. I had many of these as a child long before I knew I couldn't. So, when I heard of flourless pancakes, I thought, "Sounds perfect!" And you WILL flip for these, whether you have celiac or not.

In a large bowl, whisk together the eggs and cornmeal. In a separate bowl, mash the bananas and stir in the crushed pecans. I put the pecans in a Ziploc bag and use a meat hammer to crush. They should be a fine texture, sort of like flour. Combine the egg mixture with the banana nut mixture until well blended.

Heat a tablespoon of coconut oil or butter in a frying pan or griddle over medium heat. Drop batter by small spoonfuls on to hot pan. I like to keep my pancakes fairly small so they'll cook more quickly and be easier to flip. I use about two tablespoons of batter for each one, which makes a around a 4-inch pancake

Cook for 1–2 minutes, then flip and cook for 1–2 minutes on the other side. Repeat with the remaining batter, greasing the pan between each pancake.

These pancakes are delicious on their own, but part of the fun is experimenting with toppings. Try chopped nuts, fresh berries, a smear of jam or maybe some peanut butter. Oh, and don't forget the syrup!

---

2 bananas

2 large eggs

½ cup fine grind cornmeal

½ cup crushed pecans

Virgin coconut oil or butter

Real maple syrup

Serves 4–6

we lucky aces
goin' thru the paces
time outside
with sunshine-y faces
stickin' with the heart racers
soul lifters
dreamliner creators
one-shot this planet takers

– jet –

4

conclusion

*Guided by mindfulness and a new,
clear direction—now what?*

Wellness is a dynamic, individual, ever-
changing, fluctuating process. We should
aim to strive for a personal harmony that
feels most authentic to us.

conclusion

It's probably fair to say that most of us would prefer a calmer, more fulfilling approach to life. There are so many things we can do and so many ways we can spend our time, but oftentimes we try to do too much. This is taking a toll on our bodies and spirit, which can lead to stress-related problems such as high blood pressure, heart disease, asthma, diabetes and other illness.[50] The bottom line is that we're burning out mentally and physically, and sacrificing what is important to us in the process.

Whether you want more vitality, more connection, more independence or more adventure, it all comes down to how you spend and value your time. Your fate is not predestined. You always have a choice. You can either fill your days living in alignment with your core values, or you can fill them with things not worthy of the time you're spending on them.

"Life is a combination of both destiny and chance. There is a little role played by our destiny, and a greater part played by our free will. It is never either this or that alone. There is not a single moment that does not have a past or that does not have a future. So, the past is destiny, the future is free will, and the present moment is so beautiful."
– Sri Sri Ravi Shankar, spiritual leader and founder of Art of Living Foundation

The present moment is in your own hands, and your future will be determined by the decisions you make today. When you neglect your needs, you put a lien on your future happiness. It is true that if we have our health, we are certainly lucky, but our successes are defined by effort. Soul pilots don't rely on chance to get to their destination. We put a lot into organization, personal goals, adequate sleep, exercise and eating fresh, whole, nutritious foods. It's a discipline that—in the long run—will make you feel pretty darn lucky.

Wellness is all around us. Everywhere. However, we have to get to know ourselves and tune in to what our bodies are telling us. We have to give ourselves some respect and love. We have to do the work and the research, but we also have to listen to our hearts. Time is life. It's up to each of us to choose how we spend it.

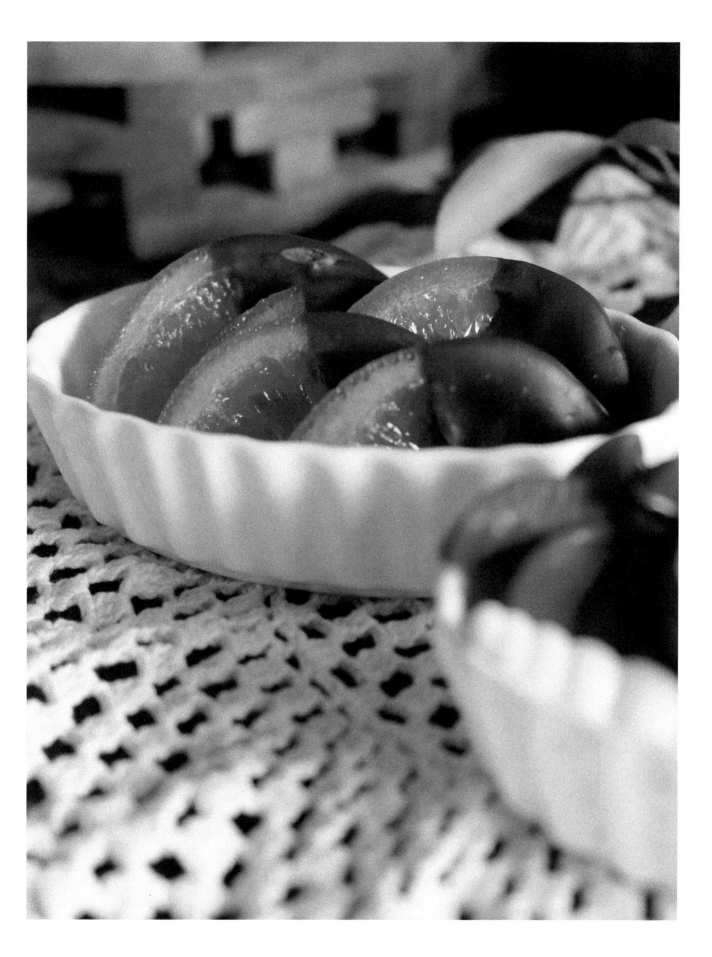

it's the people
that keep me intoxicated with life
their unconditional love high-fives
natural belly laughs
that can't be contrived
wake-up happy to be alive
feeling tall enough
to jump and touch the ceiling
true heart not concealing
happy to be healthy AF feeling!

– jet –

(5)

acknowledgments

For all that has been, thank you.
For all that is to come... yes!

This book has been a shared journey with
a number of people—both directly and
indirectly—each with their own set of life
lessons, bright insight, magic and wisdom.

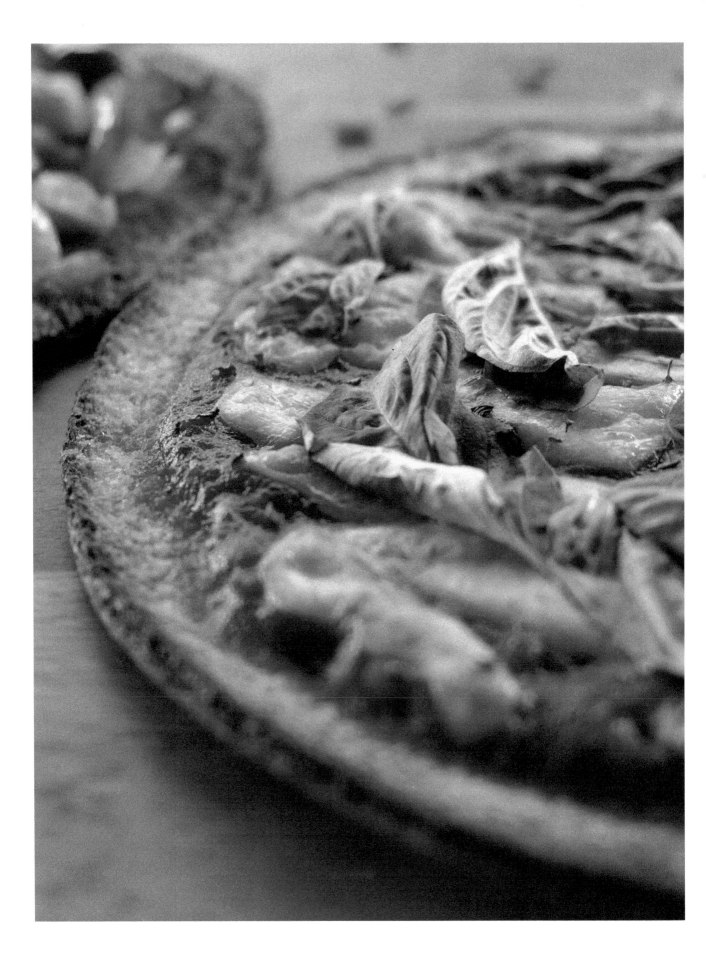

acknowledgments

When I approached Kristen Alden with the idea to turn my blog into a book, I had a very different idea of what this would look like. I thought it would be a collection of significant posts that would provide insight into the gluten-free diet. But as we began writing, this turned out to be so much more. It became a guidebook for living a mindful, healthy, authentic and inspired life—whether one has a food-related illness or not.

This isn't a complete reference guide to living with celiac disease, but there's no way it could be. There are already so many wonderful resources written about the gluten-free lifestyle such as *Gluten Is My Bitch* by April Peveteaux, *Wheat Belly* by Dr. William Davis, *The Primal Blueprint* by Mark Sisson, and *Jennifer's Way* by actress Jennifer Esposito. There's nothing we could say that they haven't said already.

Making magic is a collective effort, and *Gluten Free Soul Pilot* wouldn't be the same without Kristen's brilliant and creative spirit, her intuition and her intelligence. Kristen and I would like to thank everyone and everything that helped in the creation of this book—whether directly or indirectly: To our families for your unconditional love, support and patience through the long days and temporary sacrifices; to all our friends who had our backs and trusted we'd eventually come out on the other side; to JKS Communications for your belief in us and our mission; to Deborah Tracey whose willingness to fly cross-country to work with us gave us a jump-start early on; to Kimberly Taylor-Pestell for your work ethic and commitment to proofread and copy edit this passion project in the final hour; to the gluten-free community and our Instagram family for your inspiring messages and encouragement; and to the unexpected and challenging times that compelled us to keep moving forward with courage and a firm belief.

We are also deeply grateful to our mentors, such as Danielle LaPorte, Brené Brown, Elizabeth Gilbert, Oprah Winfrey and Marie Forleo. Your bravery, creativity and empathy lights us up and inspires us to teach more Soul Pilots how to live and lead as brilliantly as you do.

"If I had more time, I would've written a shorter letter."
– Blaise Pascal, mathematician, physicist, inventor, and writer

Thank you! Let your soul be your pilot. xoxo.

you're as important as oxygen
where do I begin
to explain your importance is endless
because you are the best
you meet the highest standards
that I possess
truly living
you stand above the rest
put my soul to the test
shooting high past the moonbeams
where your true importance
and my high standards
meet in a sweet dream

– jet –

6

references

*The smart, talented experts & influencers
who are soul pilots in their own right.*

We are indebted to the work of many
thoughtful scholars and thought leaders whose
research and sagaciousness help shape our
own philosophies and keep our spirits strong.

references

Introduction

1 "Celiac Disease Facts and Figures." The University of Chicago Medicine Celiac Disease Center. Accessed July 25, 2018. http://www.uchospitals.edu/pdf/uch_007937.pdf.

2 Davis, William. *Wheat Belly: Lose the Wheat, Lose the Weight, and Find Your Path Back to Health*. First Edition. (New York: Rodale, 2011), 92.

3 "Long-term Health Conditions." n.d. Celiac Disease Foundation. Accessed July 25, 2018. https://celiac.org/celiac-disease/understanding-celiac-disease-2/what-is-celiac-disease/24477-2/.

Flight Plan: Choose Your Destination

4 Steakley, Lia. "Why Establishing a Health Baseline is a 'Critical Starting Point for Achieving Future Health Goals.'" Stanford Medicine. January 27, 2015. https://scopeblog.stanford.edu/2015/01/27/why-establishing-a-health-baseline-is-a-critical-starting-point-for-achieving-future-health-goals/.

5 Sandelowski, Margarete, Brenda DeVellis, and Marci Campbell. "Variations in Meanings of the Personal Core Value 'Health.'" *Patient Education and Counseling* 73.2 (November 2008): 347–353. *PMC*. Accessed August 20, 2018. https://www.ncbi.nlm.nih.gov/pmc/articles/PMC2633415/.

Flight Plan: Flight Route

6 TapRooT® is a systematic process, software, and training used by leading companies around the world to investigate and fix the root causes of problems. These include major accidents, everyday incidents, minor near-misses, quality issues, human errors, maintenance problems, medical mistakes, productivity issues, manufacturing mistakes, environmental releases … in other words, all types of mission-critical problems. Taproot.com. http://www.taproot.com/archives/37771.

Flight Plan: Timeline

7 Lally, Phillippa and Benjamin Gardner. "Does intrinsic motivation strengthen physical activity habit? Modeling relationships between self-determination, past behaviour, and habit

strength." *Journal of Behavioral Medicine*. (October 2013): 488-97. Accessed August 23, 2018. https://www.ncbi.nlm.nih.gov/pubmed/22760451.

8 Lally, Phillippa and Benjamin Gardner. "Promoting habit formation." *Health Psychology Review*. (November 2010): S137–152. Accessed August 23, 2018. https://www.researchgate.net/publication/230576970_Promoting_habit_formation.

9 Jeremy Dean. *Making Habits, Breaking Habits: Why We Do Things, Why We Don't, and How to Make Any Change Stick*. First Edition. (Boston: Da Capo Press, 2013), 5–6.

10 Gardner, Benjamin, Phillippa Lally, and Jane Wardle. "Making Health Habitual: The Psychology of 'habit-Formation' and General Practice." *The British Journal of General Practice*. (December 2012): 664–666. *PMC*. Accessed August 30, 2018. https://www.ncbi.nlm.nih.gov/pmc/articles/PMC3505409/.

11 Cialdini, Robert. *Pre-suasion*. (New York, New York: Simon & Schuster, 2016), Accessed August 30, 2018. http://www.routineexcellence.com/psychology-of-habits-form-habits-make-stick/.

Flight Plan: Fuel Calculation

12 "Sleepiness May Impair the Brain's Inhibitory Control When Viewing High-calorie Foods." *Science Daily*. (June 2011). American Academy of Sleep Medicine. Accessed August 24, 2018. http://www.sciencedaily.com/releases/2011/06/110613093458.htm.

13 "The Best Diet: Quality Counts." n.d. The Nutrition Source. Harvard Health. Accessed August 24, 2018. https://www.hsph.harvard.edu/nutritionsource/healthy-weight/best-diet-quality-counts/#ref23.

14 Gardner, Meryl, Brian Wansink, Junyong Kim, and Se-Bum Park (2014). "Better Moods for Better Eating?: How Mood Influences Food Choice." *Journal of Consumer Psychology*. (July 2014): 320-335. Accessed September 02, 2018. https://www.sciencedirect.com/science/article/abs/pii/S1057740814000060.

15 Hartman, Lauren R. "The Role of Sensory Properties in Food Development." Food Processing. July 27, 2016. Accessed September 02, 2018. http://www.foodprocessing.com/articles/2016/sensory-properties-in-food-development/?start=0.

16 Verloigne, Maïté et al. "Self-Determined Motivation towards Physical Activity in Adolescents Treated for Obesity: An Observational Study." *The International Journal of Behavioral Nutrition and Physical Activity*. (September 2011): 97. *PMC*. Accessed September 09 2018. https://www.ncbi.nlm.nih.gov/pubmed/21923955.

Flight Plan: Air Traffic Compliance

17 Breines Juliana G. and Serena Chen. "Self-compassion increases self-improvement motivation." *Personality and Social Psychology Bulletin: SAGE Journals.* (May 2012): 1133-43. Accessed September 08, 2018. http://journals.sagepub.com/doi/abs/10.1177/0146167212445599.

18 Neff, Kristin D. "Self-compassion: An Alternative Conceptualization of a Healthy Attitude Toward Oneself." *Psychology Press.* (September 2010): 85–101. Accessed September 10, 2018. https://self-compassion.org/wp-content/uploads/publications/SCtheoryarticle.pdf.

19 Neff, Kristin D. "Self-compassion, Self-esteem, and Well-being. *Social and Personality Psychology Compass.* (2011): 1–12. Accessed September 10, 2018. https://self-compassion.org/wp-content/uploads/2015/12/SC.SE_.Well-being.pdf.

20 Fredrickson, Barbara L. "The Role of Positive Emotions in Positive Psychology: The Broaden-and-Build Theory of Positive Emotions." *The American Psychologist.* (March 2001): 218–226. Accessed September 10, 2018. https://www.ncbi.nlm.nih.gov/pmc/articles/PMC3122271/.

21 "Cognitive Behavioral Therapy." Informed Health Online [Internet]. Last Update: September 8, 2016. Accessed September 12, 2018. https://www.ncbi.nlm.nih.gov/pubmedhealth/PMH0072481/.

22 Manghani, Kishu. "Quality Assurance: Importance of Systems and Standard Operating Procedures." *Perspectives in Clinical Research.* (January-March 2011): 34–37. PMC. Accessed September 14, 2018. https://www.ncbi.nlm.nih.gov/pmc/articles/PMC3088954/.

Flight Plan: Arrival

23 Karolinska Institutet. "Everyday Exercise Has Surprisingly Positive Health Benefits." *Science Daily.* January 25, 2018. http://www.sciencedaily.com/releases/2018/01/180125110030.htm.

24 Krakovsky, Marina. "The Effort Effect". *Stanford Magazine.* March/April 2007 Issue. https://alumni.stanford.edu/get/page/magazine/article/?article_id=32124.

25 Amabile, Teresa and Steven J. Kramer. "The Power of Small Wins." *Harvard Business Review.* May 2011 Issue. https://hbr.org/2011/05/the-power-of-small-wins.

26 Sansone, Randy A. and Lori A. Sansone. "Gratitude and Well Being: The Benefits of Appreciation." *Psychiatry MMC.* (November 2010): 18–22. Accessed September 22, 2018. https://www.ncbi.nlm.nih.gov/pmc/articles/PMC3010965/.

27 Robbins, Mel. "Why Motivation Is Garbage," filmed July 2017, Impact Theory video, 49:54, https://impacttheory.com/blog/why-motivation-is-garbage/.

28 Rock, David. "New Study Shows Humans Are on Autopilot Nearly Half the Time."

Psychology Today. November 14, 2010. https://www.psychologytoday.com/us/blog/your-brain-work/201011/new-study-shows-humans-are-autopilot-nearly-half-the-time.

The Four Principles

29 Armenta, Christina, Katherine Jacobs Bao, Sonja Lyubomirsky, and Kennon M. Sheldon. "Is Lasting Change Possible? Lessons from the Hedonistic Adaptation Prevention Model." *Stability of Happiness*. First Edition. (San Diego: Elsevier, 2014), 57–74.

The Four Principles (Knowledge): Single-ingredient Simplicity

30 Cordain, Loren et al. "Origins and Evolution of the Western Diet: Health Implications for the 21st Century." *The American Journal of Clinical Nutrition*, Volume 81, Issue 2, (February 2005): 341–354. Accessed May 25, 2018. https://academic.oup.com/ajcn/article/81/2/341/4607411.

The Four Principles (Knowledge): Easy New Year's Resolution: Water

31 LaMotte, Sandee. "Are You Drinking Enough Water to Be Healthy?" CNN. September 28, 2017. Accessed October 08, 2018. https://www.cnn.com/2017/09/27/health/benefits-of-water-and-fluids/index.html.

32 "Food Composition Databases Show Foods List." USDA Food Composition Databases. Accessed October 08, 2018. https://ndb.nal.usda.gov/ndb/foods/.

The Four Principles (Knowledge): Cooking With Unconscious Competence

33 "The Conscious Competence Ladder: Keeping Going When Learning Gets Tough." Groupthink - Decision Making Skills Training from MindTools.com. Accessed October 08, 2018. https://www.mindtools.com/pages/article/newISS_96.htm.

The Four Principles (Knowledge): You're Sweet Enough Already

34 Jones, Daniel. 2017. "Your Starbucks Drink Is like Eating 7 Doughnuts, Study Says." New York Post. *New York Post*. November 10, 2017. https://nypost.com/2017/11/09/your-starbucks-drink-is-like-eating-7-doughnuts-study-says/.

35 Davis, William. 2014. "Don't Fall for 'Gluten-Free' Foods Made with Junk Carbs." Dr. William Davis. July 22, 2014. https://www.wheatbellyblog.com/2014/07/dont-fooled-gluten-free-foods/.

36 Fleming, Amy. 2014. "Mindfulness or Cake? The Battle against Stress and Comfort-Eating." *The Guardian*. Guardian News and Media. July 1, 2014. https://www.theguardian.com/.

lifeandstyle/wordofmouth/2014/jul/01/mindfulness-cake-stress-comfort-eating-obesity-heart-disease-type-2-diabetes-ban-sugar.

37   Price, Annie. n.d. "Benefits of Dark Chocolate You Won't Believe." DrAxe.com. Accessed October 10, 2018. https://draxe.com/benefits-of-dark-chocolate/.

The Four Principles (Strength): Stay Positive While Going Negative

38   Zelman, Kathleen M. "6 Steps to Changing Bad Eating Habits." WebMD. Accessed October 08, 2018. https://www.webmd.com/diet/obesity/features/6-steps-to-changing-bad-eating-habits#1.

The Four Principles (Strength): Your Vibe Attracts Your Tribe

39   Wright, Karen. "Authentic and Eudaimonic." *Psychology Today*. Accessed October 09, 2018. https://www.psychologytoday.com/us/articles/200805/authentic-and-eudaimonic?amp.

The Four Principles (Strength): Asset-based Thinking

40   Cramer, Kathy. Asset Based Thinking. The Cramer Institute. Accessed October 08, 2018. https://cramerinstitute.com/asset-based-thinking/.

The Four Principles (Strength): Make Your Own 7-Minute Workout

41   Yeager, Selene. "Exercise: The Least You Can Do." Oprah.com. Accessed October 08, 2018. http://www.oprah.com/health/even-10-minutes-of-exercise-a-day-can-improve-health.

The Four Principles (Wisdom): Rock-solid (and Fragile) Foundation

42   *The Seattle Times*. Accessed October 08, 2018. http://old.seattletimes.com/special/mlk/king/words/blueprint.html.

The Four Principles (Wisdom): Advice To My Younger Self

43   "Symptoms, Diagnosis and Treatment | NIH MedlinePlus the Magazine." n.d. *MedlinePlus*. U.S. National Library of Medicine. Accessed October 10, 2018. https://medlineplus.gov/magazine/issues/spring15/articles/spring15pg4.html.

44   "Celiac Disease and Lactose Intolerance." n.d. Beyond Celiac. Accessed October 10, 2018. https://www.beyondceliac.org/celiac-disease/related-conditions/lactose-intolerance/.

45 "Connection Between Mental and Physical Health." n.d. CMHA Ontario. Accessed October 10, 2018. https://ontario.cmha.ca/documents/connection-between-mental-and-physical-health/.

The Four Principles (Wisdom): Walk With the Dreamers

46 "Celiac Disease Triggers." 2016. Amy Burkhart M.D., R.D. May 17, 2016. Accessed October 10, 2018. http://theceliacmd.com/2014/09/triggers-celiac-disease-one-possible-answer/.

47 "Celiac Disease Support Groups." n.d. Beyond Celiac. Accessed October 10, 2018. https://www.beyondceliac.org/celiac-disease/additional-information/support-groups/.

48 "Celiac Disease Runs in Families." n.d. Beyond Celiac. Accessed October 10, 2018. https://www.beyondceliac.org/celiac-disease/family-testing/.

The Four Principles (Inspiration): Catalyst for Happiness

49 Gilbert, Dan. "The Surprising Science of Happiness," filmed February 2004, TED video, 21:01, https://www.ted.com/talks/dan_gilbert_asks_why_are_we_happy?language=en.

The Four Principles (Inspiration): Disconnect to Reconnect

50 Swartzberg, John. "Walking in Nature." *Berkeley Wellness*. December 1, 2010. http://www.berkeleywellness.com/healthy-mind/stress/article/walking-woods.

Page 141 Photo courtesy of Mark Widick, markwidick.com.

Conclusion

51 Salleh, MR. "Life Event, Stress and Illness." *The Malaysian Journal of Medical Sciences*. Accessed October 11, 2018. https://www.ncbi.nlm.nih.gov/pmc/articles/PMC3341916/.

about the authors

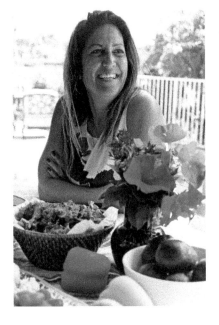

jet widick

Jet Widick is a poet, former nurse and founder of *Gluten Free Sage*, a wellness blog that promotes the power of perspective and the ability to heal through a healthful lifestyle and artful experiences. Poetry has always been an essential part of Jet's life, but it wasn't until her celiac diagnosis—after 15 years of living with a mystery illness—when she discovered how emotional strength and good health can open up one's world to inspiration and desire, both which propel a person into the realm of possibility and shift the way we perceive our own capabilities. Her sons gave her the nickname Jet (short for Jeanette) which embodies her wellness journey, fueled by her love of nature and taking off with tremendous creative energy and vitality.

kristen alden

Kristen Alden is an independent creative consultant, artist and graphic designer with over 15 years' experience in broadcasting, marketing and communications, and brand development for nonprofits, small businesses and entrepreneurs. Throughout her years as a creative and communications expert, her passion for health and wellness has inspired her to be a part of projects whose missions were to help others better themselves. Kristen believes that great design has the power to educate, inspire and ignite change. When she's not fastidiously creating with her collaborators, you can find her far away from the computer developing a vision for the everyday and an organized way of making things more beautiful.

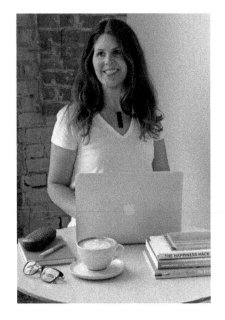

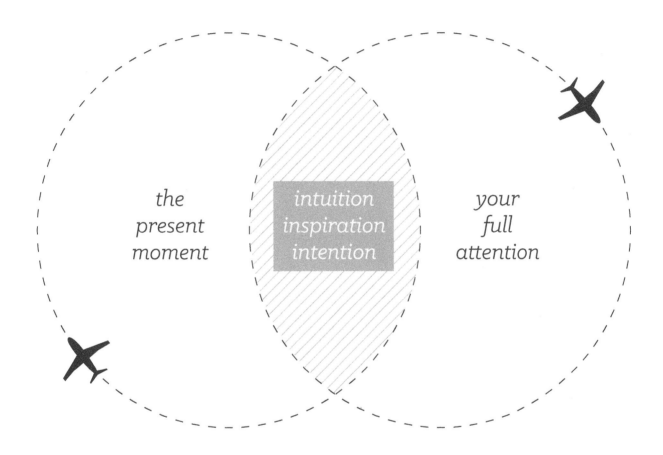

CPSIA information can be obtained
at www.ICGtesting.com
Printed in the USA
LVHW011215270623
750925LV00009B/527